# Gas and Air

Tales of Pregnancy, Birth and Beyond

# Gas and Air

Tales of Pregnancy, Birth and Beyond

An anthology edited by
Jill Dawson and Margo Daly

BLOOMSBURY

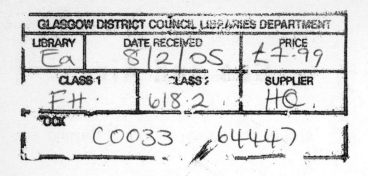
First published in Great Britain 2002

Copyright © 2002 in the edition and the Introduction: Jill Dawson and
Margo Daly. Each contribution shall remain the copyright of the contributor

The moral rights of the authors have been asserted

Bloomsbury Publishing Plc, 38 Soho Square, London W1D 3HB

A CIP catalogue record is available from the British Library

ISBN 0 7475 5823 X

10 9 8 7 6 5 4 3 2 1

Typeset by Hewer Text Ltd, Edinburgh
Printed in Great Britain by Clays Ltd, St Ives plc

For our children: Lila, Lewis and Felix

# CONTENTS

# Introduction

*'Birth, and copulation and death. That's all the facts, when you come to brass tacks.'*

T.S. Eliot

Literature seems to have the other two – copulation and death – pretty well covered, but gets a little sketchy when it comes to birth. Until recently, fathers were excluded from witnessing or participating in the experience of giving birth, so I suppose we should not be too surprised if serious literature by men has either avoided, marginalised or sentimentalised the subject. But then women writers have not necessarily redressed the balance either. This might well be because so many great women writers of the past were childless: Virginia Woolf, Jane Austen, Emily Dickinson and Simone de Beauvoir spring readily to mind. Perhaps it is also due to the difficulties that birth, the most animal, primal and *visceral* of experiences, presents to those wanting to pin it down in language. But writers love to rise to such a challenge, to find words for the unsayable; that's what they *do*. One can only assume that most significant of all has been a residual taboo surrounding the most female of experiences.

Much has changed in the last thirty years. For one thing, 95 per cent of fathers (in the UK) now opt to be at the birth of their child. For another, our knowledge and under-standing of birth and pregnancy has made phenomenal progress. We now take it for granted, for instance, that we can see and hear our baby in the womb and even take home a 'photograph' of him or her. The number of women who manage to have a family and write for a living has significantly increased; hardly surprising then that the experience of having children often becomes the subject of the writing. Birth as a literary experience is now firmly on the map.

It was the extraordinarily moving account by Peter Carey of his son's birth, addressed to his child, which inspired this anthology. My co-editor, Margo, and I were both pregnant, and in email correspondence with each other (she had newly returned to Sydney; I had recently moved to the Fens). The beauty and detail in Carey's piece is affecting and unusual; it becomes even more so when you are pregnant. This alteration in consciousness is part of the folklore of pregnancy but one which both Margo and I found to be true! As the protagonist of Emily Perkins's story *Little Hearts* says of her yoga classes with the orange candles and tapes with crashing waves and seagull sounds: 'I am pregnant and my tolerance for certain things has mysteriously expanded.'

Initially, we were aiming at a pregnant reader (or expectant father) in putting together this anthology. Margo and I had both discovered a sudden and insatiable appetite to read more and more about pregnancy, birth and babies which accompanied our growing bulk. We eagerly exchanged discoveries: Julie Myerson's pregnant heroine, in her novel *Sleepwalking*, embarking on a sexy affair, or Susan Johnson's terrifying account in her book *A Better Woman* of just what labour can do to a woman's body. In the main, though, manuals and *How To . . .* books vastly outnumber works of fiction on the subject, which is what persuaded us to gather together the stories collected here.

I didn't even have the excuse for my mania of it being a first-time pregnancy, as Margo did. When I was first pregnant, over a decade ago, I can't remember reading anything much about pregnancy, birth or parenthood. I was twenty-six years old and the only one in my circle of friends who had any intention, desire or interest in having a child. I didn't join a National Childbirth class or attend yoga classes or write a birth plan. In fact, like many women the world over, I was convinced that pregnancy is not actually a very big deal.

Second time around, things couldn't have been more different. I'd been alerted to the unexpected; all the things which could go wrong, all the ways in which the experience defied and surpassed my expectations of it. I decided to be a little better prepared. My matter-of-fact attitude of old resurfaced occasionally during the editing of this book – and I believe it is the better for it! – but in the main I was far more interested in what was happening to me this time.

I wonder if the change in me – and our joint craving to read about birth and babies – reflects a corresponding change in Western attitudes towards pregnancy and birth. Huge media attention in the last few years has been paid to glamorous celebrity mothers like Madonna, Posh Spice and Catherine Zeta-Jones. Suddenly pregnancy is sexy. Birth and babies are big news, at least for a short while. Having a child is actually seen as a significant event, rather than the non-event that its marginal place in literature might previously have implied. Maybe we were simply sensitive to external influences and approbation of the choices we'd made. Incidentally, a media delight in photographing pregnant celebrities has not extended to any new attitudes towards women's bodies in general. Breasts, I've noticed, are still always shown as sexy and decorative, and breast-feeding remains a largely hidden area of public life.

As Margo and I shared details of our pregnancies and

the arrival of our new children on both sides of the globe, our experiences seemed at times highly individual and unique; at others, of course, quotidian and universal. This collection, being individual stories by some marvellous contemporary writers, attempts to capture that dichotomy. We gave our writers the theme as their starting point and then left them to get on with it.

The collection contains memoirs mingled in with short stories and extracts. After some discussion, we have chosen not to indicate which inclusions are autobiographical and which are fiction, preferring to leave work to speak for itself. We enjoyed the blurring of the boundaries between fiction and memoir: it seemed particularly relevant to the subject-matter. Some writers naturally enough wanted to protect their children from too close an association with the piece included, others only felt liberated when they could come clean and write passionately of their own experiences. We hope this opens, rather than closes, the possible interpretations of the tales.

This is a contemporary collection about birth. Julia Darling's protagonist tells us: 'I got the sperm through a self-help group. I administered it with a cake icing syringe.' There are plenty of single mothers, Caesarean deliveries and fathers' perspectives. But the collection also contains material some readers might find uncomfortable: stillbirths, unwanted pregnancies, post-natal depression, autism. When I was given a one in three chance of having a child with Down's syndrome as part of my ante-natal screening, I suddenly noticed how worryingly lacking in useful information all the birth manuals were on so many things about pregnancy which really matter. We've tried to avoid that pitfall. We've included much that's wondrous, much that's joyous, ecstatic – along with much that's ordinary. We've included, after thinking long and hard about it, Hannah Fink's moving story about a stillbirth. We want to add as a postscript the fact that as we write this, Hannah has recently given birth to a baby girl. For me, Kathy Page's simplicity sums up the experience best: 'moving on, but at the same time going back, where everyone has been before'.

*Jill Dawson*

Unlike Jill, I was to be totally prepared for the birth of my first baby. There was the weekly yoga workout, the antenatal classes and the parenting course at my hospital, the visits to the midwives at the birthing centre there, where I planned to have a waterbirth, the constant referring to not only the Kitzinger bible but also Penelope Leach and Janet Balaskas (the UK trio of gurus), the Australian Kaz Cooke's irreverent manual *The Real Guide to Pregnancy* and that American classic *What to Expect When You're Expecting*. (What I didn't expect, and refused to even consider, was that I might have to have a Caesarean.) When watching television or a film at the cinema, any reference to or depiction of pregnancy, birth or babies had me fully alert and fixated to the screen, taking in all the details. This and a finely honed radar for any other pregnant women in the vicinity reminded me of the childhood obsession with other children: the similar delighted response to child characters on screen, and the engrossed appraisal of any other new child in sight, which I see now with my own baby, instinctively looking for her kind. TV news stories of the floods in Mozambique and a woman giving birth in a tree, high above the raging waters, had me transfixed and weeping.

Similarly, as a voracious reader of fiction, I was fascinated when I stumbled across pregnant characters or birth scenes, and I thought back to other examples I'd read in the past. Pregnant characters were often tragic, often written by men. Births weren't really described but were generally a plot device for the woman to die, or at least become very ill. I remembered the line from Shakespeare's *Macbeth*; the play's most graphic description of a Caesarean, which later repeated through my head: Macduff 'from his mother's womb untimely ripped'. I thought of Hetty Sorrel, the farm girl seduced and then abandoned by an aristocrat and on the road alone, desperately seeking him in the final weeks of her pregnancy, in George Eliot's *Adam Bede* (1859); the deserted pregnant wife Yvonne de Galais in *Le Grand Meaulnes* by Alain-Fournier (1913); Tolstoy's *Anna Karenina* (1876) and the child she bears to her lover Count Bronsky, nearly dying in the process; the protagonist in Penelope Mortimer's *The Pumpkin Eater* (1962), who is obsessed with being pregnant and having yet more babies; the young incest victim, Celie, pregnant in the opening pages of *The Color Purple* by Alice Walker (1983); Nora Ephron's wisecracking Rachel, a pregnant cookery writer, dumped by her Washington newspaper columnist husband in *Heartburn* (1983); Harriet Lovatt in Doris Lessing's *The Fifth Child* (1988), when her fifth pregnancy, and the resulting child, the strange Ben, wrecks her happy home.

Of these, I found I identified most with Rachel of *Heartburn*, seven months' pregnant and rueing the fact that she couldn't exactly throw herself into the dating scene: she was funny but also more vulnerable emotionally and physically than she could ever be again. Similarly, when compiling this collection, I particularly identified with the women going it alone: Julia Darling's story *Pearl*, or Alice Jerome's *Gwendolyn* and Nikki Gemmell's *Tales of the Recent Past*. These stories especially and the two which included Caesareans – *Gwendolyn* and Eva Sallis's *The 'Kursk'* – confirmed that my feelings, my anxieties and fears weren't unusual, that I was not alone.

When my breech baby refused to turn, and was found to have a head larger than normal, I agreed to have an elective Caesarean. Greedy for experience, to know every single thing about life, I cried because I wouldn't feel the 'pangs' of childbirth, not a single contraction. I may never know what that is like, but these stories give me some idea: 'I am heaving between the waves of pain, waiting, angling to face the next. Each wave must be taken as a right angle, cleft with the smooth deep V of my breastbone, my head calm and still' (Eva Sallis). Or Julia Darling: 'That night my contractions start. They are like cart-horses galloping through my body.'

Nor did I experience my waters breaking, though the event in Simone Lazaroo's story, on the white tiles of a department store's fast-food basement, was my greatest fear in the final weeks.

That other moment, which starts the whole scary ball rolling – conception – many people can't pinpoint. Two stories in this collection capture very romantic moments. As Peter Carey's wife gives birth to their son: 'We kissed with soft passionate lips as we did the day we lay on the bed at Lovett Bay and conceived you. That day the grass outside the window was a brilliant green beneath the vibrant petals of fallen jacaranda.' And in Rosie Waitt's story at Undara: 'I remember the feel of the stone, the 300-million-year-old pink granite, how special it seemed . . . Then, while the children slept above and the rain pelted around us, our baby was conceived.'

The vividness of my own pregnancy had begun to wear off through the editing stages, but each story brought back strong feelings and sensations. There are exultant images: 'The sight of the umbilical cord, glorious in its violent colours, like something washed up on a beach, still pulsing with the salty green trace of the sea' (Jill Dawson) and simple but profound revelations. Rosie Waitt on the road with husband and two daughters in an unforgiving Australian outback, has a near-miss car accident: 'Suddenly I feel very vulnerable. I want to cry because I could have the baby at any time and we are a long way from anywhere and I don't want my baby to be born out here.'

For all the advanced technological help on offer, birth can still be dangerous stuff, particularly when help is not at hand. David Guterson gives us a glimpse of the doctor's perspective in the extract from *East of the Mountains*, where a retired family doctor is required to attend an emergency birth, the first he's dealt with in over forty years. Any number of yoga classes, Active Birth classes and plans for home delivery and waterbeds won't guarantee the labour you want. Judith Bryan in *Deliverance* describes learning the hard lesson to take nothing for granted. Modern women, used to being in control of their bodies and their lives, must now bow to a greater will, that of a new life struggling to be born. Whether or not the experience meets our high and often romantic expectations, we can at least hope to emerge with dignity, pride – and our child intact.

*Margo Daly*

# Little Hearts

## *Emily Perkins*

It was maybe a full minute before I realised I was stuck. The egg was still in my hand, and my hand was still poised over the edge of the bowl. I was frozen, certain that I couldn't crack the egg without smashing it so shell and goo went everywhere. Butter and sugar, flecked with black specks of vanilla stick, lay all plumped and creamy in the bowl. It was time for the next step. The oven clock's sticky red second hand ticked. Eventually I managed to put the egg down on the bench without breaking it and went to the sofa, where I curled up in the same position the baby had been in last time I looked. We had had a scan a month earlier, the twenty-week scan where they tell you if the foetus has spina bifida or not. Our baby was normal. We were relieved, though I suppose I would have loved it just as much if it were not. As I lay on the sofa I could feel it flutter and push at my insides. It was still an it: we had asked not to be told the sex.

Michael was out late, providing for our future. He was exceptionally good at this, which was one of the many things I found sexy about him. The cake was meant to be a nice, wifely surprise, but it looked as though I was going to have to put on special underwear instead. My mother deeply disapproves of the kind of woman I am. The kind she has struggled so hard, in recent years, not to be. Don't misunderstand me – there was nothing ironic about the cake gesture. I absolutely wanted Michael to come home to the warm, inviting smell of baking; I wanted everything here to be appealing, smooth, calm. It was just that I couldn't seem to crack the egg.

The night before, we'd been at a dinner party hosted by Sam and Eloise. Everyone was drunk, except me. The starter had been poached scallops and the main course was a blue-cheese roulade, neither of which I was allowed to eat in case I gave the baby salmonella, or listeria, I could never remember which. I snuck downstairs into the basement kitchen to stuff some extra bread in my mouth. Sam and Eloise's place was vast, and their kitchen walls were lime-washed plaster and their whiteware wasn't white but made of brushed stainless steel, great iceberg objects humming down there in the dark. From upstairs came the muffled sound of laughter, and I wondered what, or who, was its cause.

We've known each other since secondary school, Eloise and I; my second secondary school. Eloise is a doctor now and Sam writes interactive dramas, so between them they have God complexes pretty much sewn up. I don't mind because my inferiority complex is the size of a barn, if that isn't too grandiose a thing to say. Perhaps a small shed. Anyway, when Eloise announces her wish that all patients would lie neatly and still in their beds wearing regulation striped pyjamas, I think she is just teasing. The fascist implications surely do not escape her; she is definitely winding us up. It works on Michael. I can almost see the words bulging from his forehead like cartoon eggs as he forces himself to keep quiet. Michael is a doctor too. He and Eloise trained together, and both made the decision to go into private practice at the same time. Michael agonised over it. Eloise did not.

You should have seen our wedding. My side all got drunk, and my mother cried for the wrong reasons. My father, I think, was drunk in the register office, and it was eleven in the morning. I was incredibly happy, happier than I had ever expected to be. I had thought being a bride would be embarrassing, everyone gawking at you, feeling like you were the only one dressed in a silly clown outfit, his ex-girlfriends whispering about your shoes. But when I saw him for the first time that day I felt a fizzing, hot rush of love and it all bubbled up to my face and I smiled like a loon and didn't stop until we were asleep that night. Maybe not even then.

We met through Eloise, at a Christmas function just after she had become a junior doctor. Michael took my phone number and called me in the new year. He wanted me to show him some art galleries. We stood outside a photographer's studio in the snow, having disagreed about everything we had seen. Pigeons burbled from under the eaves of a building that was nothing more than a burnt-out shell. The artist had given us apple brandy to drink. The street, the snowy cars, the grime-littered doorways were all black and white, sooty; the sky was like a stretch of dirty muslin over slate. I hadn't understood the last three things Michael had said. He was scowling. 'Do you go through life thinking all conversation has to be this hard?' I asked him. The frown broke and he smiled, and it was as though I'd been given a prize, the best prize, and for no reason.

I would like to create a secret, fairy-tale bedroom, with twirling glimmers of light, and jewel-coloured glass, and music boxes and friendly shadows. Stars on the ceiling, mermaids on the wall. For the baby, I mean. Of course for the baby.

It is nearly the end of my weekly ante-natal yoga session. I belong to a class of twelve women, all of us at varying stages of pregnancy, who meet each Thursday morning to be guided through breathing and stretching exercises. The room we meet in is on the top floor of a community centre in our pleasant and affluent suburb. Leafy branches blow about just outside the window, and this, combined with the wooden floors and bare walls, gives you the feeling of being in a tree hut. What's the password? I don't know. Mostly we swap stories of sleepless nights and lower leg cramps, unpredictable bladders and swollen fingers. Gold bands cut into the newly fleshy bits between our knuckles. I think everybody at yoga has a wedding ring.

It is hard to shake the feeling that all of these women have done it before, although this is a first-time mothers' class and we are equally uninitiated. Perhaps it is just me who feels I haven't been let in on the secret. Our yoga tutor, Paula, is a wide-hipped, reassuringly stern woman with rampant red hair. She had her babies years and years ago, but seems to remember just what it was like and talks us through our poses in a low, calm voice. 'Feel the baby,' she murmurs, 'feel the baby rocking.' Under Paula's sensible gaze we don't give in to the urge to compare bumps and estimated due dates; we don't stare at Caroline's increasingly downy cheeks or snicker when Harriet farts getting into the dog pose. We are well behaved.

This Thursday morning in late spring is especially sunny. Light gleams from the leaves on the plane trees as they brush against each other in the breeze. Paula is burning an orange candle and her tape plays seagull and crashing waves sounds. At any previous time in my life I would have snorted at this, but I am pregnant and my tolerance for certain things has mysteriously expanded. We are all shuffling around to get our blankets and pull on socks for the relaxation session, during which at least four of us will fall asleep and Judy the American will begin to snore.

I can never properly relax during these sessions, no matter how convincing Paula's words are when she says, 'Let go, release, let go.' The room is too full of women. I have just lain down and am twitching my too-small blanket over me – everything is too small now, my clothes, towels, bedding – and trying to settle the lavender-scented eye-bag over my closed lids, when the door at the other end of the room creaks open and I hear a woman's voice. I know the voice. It's been fifteen years since I heard it, but I know the voice.

Now I am in the organic grocer's down the street from the community centre and a man with dreadlocks is asking me if I am all right. I'm standing in a corner, behind a plastic stand containing different varieties of bread. I'm cold. 'Yes, fine thanks,' I say to the man, and pick up a rye and sunflower-seed loaf to take with me to the counter. My fingers are numb, and I struggle to find the right change. When I emerge into the day I have to pause for a moment to get my bearings. This is my village, these are my local shops, there is the park and up the hill is my house. I can definitely get up the hill to my house. The streets are flooded with sunshine. I scan the footpaths for that face I have not seen in fifteen years. People come and go, attached to pushchairs and car-keys and paper bags full of food. I hold my shoulder bag and my loaf of bread tight to me. An elderly man, picking his way along with a cane. I fall into step between him and the wrought-iron tables of women nattering over late-morning caffe latte. Still she does not show herself. A group of boys overtake the old man. I hurry to keep pace with them, hiding behind their rowdy laughter, along the road and up the footpath where it becomes steeper. The boys' chatter drowns out the sound of any footsteps following me.

At the gate to my house I break off from them and run to

my door, fumbling amongst all the receipts and lipstick and nail files and crap in my bag for the keys. The key, I jab the key at the lock, fingers thick and clumsy. I glance back again but can't even focus properly to see if she's there, then at last the key fits. I let myself in as fast as I can and shut the door. The hall unfolds in front of me, and the stairs are quiet, and the doors into all the other rooms are closed. To my left, the telephone hangs on the wall, silent. I remember silences. Breathing. Threats.

Later, while Michael is standing at the kitchen bench shaving pecorino into the rocket salad, I drink some wine and try to remember what had been said. Paula had started off brusque, angry that her relaxation session was being interrupted. 'We're busy in here,' she had said. 'Are you waiting for the next class?'

'I think I'm terribly late for this class,' said Christine, for it was unmistakably Christine, that deep delivery, those certain consonants and precise vowels. 'There's been a bomb scare and the traffic from town is murder. Then I couldn't get a parking space. Have I missed everything?'

This, I think while Michael is trying to crack fresh macadamia nuts from their shells, was typical Christine: unflustered, unhurried, direct. She can instantly make anyone feel that they are in the wrong.

'No,' Paula had said, 'well yes, we're just coming to the relaxing bit now. I'm sorry. Why don't you take off your shoes and lie down? We'll talk at the end of the class about next week.'

If I had been late, if I had been stuck in traffic and then unable to find a parking space, I don't think I'd have made it up the stairs and through the doors into a room full of strange women. 'What are you doing?' I ask Michael as he enters the kitchen with a hammer in his hand. I hadn't noticed that he had been gone.

'Bastards won't crack,' he says, raising the heavy metal

head over the woody marbles of macadamias. 'Tough little fuckers, aren't you?'

I met Eloise in town for coffee, and was feeling very large. When it came time to pay I caused a gridlock in the patisserie doorway. The skin above my stomach was sore from being stretched, though there were no silver lightning streaks across it yet. I sat on the bus home, a white box, prettily tied with a gold ribbon, on my lap. The cake inside was almond and apple, Michael's favourite. My pulse was racing slightly from the coffee and I was feeling guilty for doing that to the baby. Some scientists did a test once on spiders, and they could still spin webs on alcohol or amphetamines, but caffeine sent them into a tangle of panic. This is the sort of fact that Michael scoffs at – the spiders panicked, he asks, or the scientists? – and I have to admit I don't remember where I read it. Maybe in a magazine at the hospital, waiting for a woman who never looked up to take my blood.

There was a woman next to me on the bus; we were sitting by the back doors on the bench seats reserved for fat pregnant ladies and old men with stained trousers. This woman wasn't pregnant. She had thick grey hair and beetley eyebrows. 'They're heart-breakers,' she said, nodding at my stomach. 'Little heart-breakers.' I smiled, and she said, 'The first time, I came to at the top of my mother's stairs and I was just in my nightdress.'

I nodded, and looked down at my hands.

'I'd been all through the town,' she said, louder, 'just in my nightdress.' The white-haired man sitting opposite me made a humphing noise.

'Because I blacked out, you see. I was just in my night-dress – I'd been wandering, unconscious.'

'Mm,' I said.

'And they don't know, the doctors can't say how I found

my way to my mother's house, how I knew where to go. I was in my nightdress and I was unconscious. It's even got the doctors confused.' The bus stopped for some traffic lights. She stood up. 'My boy, he was only three weeks old when they took him away and I never heard nothing. Not even a Christmas card.'

I checked. She wasn't looking at me.

'They knew where to write to me but I never heard nothing.' The bus jerked into motion and she sat down again. 'Not even a Christmas card,' she said, in a quieter voice. That was all. The brows came down; her face shut in on itself.

'Eloise said if she was having a baby she'd have a voluntary C-section,' I told Michael.

He looked up from the *British Medical Journal* and opened his mouth as if he was going to say something, then shut it. After a moment he asked, 'What do you want?'

'Just to have it normally, if I can.'

'Well, then.'

All of a sudden I didn't want to be discussing this any more. 'Shall we go to the movies this weekend?'

'When did you talk to Eloise?'

'I met her this morning.'

'Oh. Yes, let's.' He turned a page of the magazine. 'Didn't you have yoga this morning?'

'I didn't go. I wasn't really in the mood.' I began to look for our copy of the *Guide*.

Later, when Michael walked past on his way to the kitchen, he squeezed my shoulder. 'You'll be great,' he said.

Michael was on nights so he couldn't come to the antenatal class at the hospital. He knows what to expect, anyway. Eloise offered to come with me but that wasn't somehow the point, so I sat through the waterbirth video on my own. When, on the television monitor, the woman in labour moaned in pain and arched her neck like a sea lion, and the underwater camera showed the baby crowning between her ghostly pale legs, every person in the room held their breath. There was another push, and a screaming roar, and the baby swam out and up to the surface of the pool. Its father scooped it into his enormous hands. My whole body felt as though it was held in a giant grip and then let go. I looked around the room at the frightened faces of the women. Perhaps we all, for a minute, felt the same way.

The phone at home used to ring every afternoon at four. After school, but before my parents were back from work. If I didn't answer it the ringing would never stop, it could go on for over an hour, and there might be knocking on the door as well, voices through the keyhole. When I did answer, there was sometimes nothing, sometimes laughter, sometimes words. *You're going to suffer. There's going to be violence, real violence, you're going to be in pain, real pain.* Sometimes the receiver at the other end would be dropped and I would listen to a staged conversation about how ugly I was, and how I smelt, and how my parents had no money and my clothes were shit.

My father worked in the same firm as her father, and if I told anyone about this, Christine said, her father would have him fired. At school it was no different. She followed me down the corridors, whispering in my ear. 'We'll get you later, I'm going to do you, I told my boyfriend's friend about you and he's going to rape you, don't you dare look at me, don't you turn around, keep walking you ugly mole, that's right, if you fucking cry you're really going to get hurt.' I would open my locker to find a used sanitary pad, a maggoty sandwich, a dead mouse. They made jokes about my name. They called me an abortion.

I don't know why it was me that this happened to, and not anybody else. Of course, after a bit, I believed it was my fault. We had moved, were new to the area, and my parents thought this expensive, exclusive school would give me the best start. Most of the other girls knew one another already and had formed cliques, but still that doesn't explain what it was that Christine saw in me, what made her do it. I was fourteen, and my body was changing so fast I didn't know who I was any more. I developed a twitch: my head jerked several times a minute in a quick, hard nod. I smiled at everyone, longing to please, desperate for friendship. I talked to nobody.

A few years ago Michael and I were at a drinks function for a sculptor I knew. We had not been together long. I was madly in love, euphoric and invulnerable. We moved about the party arm in arm, knocking back champagne even though Michael was on call. In those days we both smoked – everybody smoked – and the room was full of hazy outlines, people looming and receding like gondoliers through fog. Somebody grabbed my elbow and I turned to see a girl who had been part of Christine's gang, a girl I hadn't seen in eleven or twelve years, beaming, shouting, 'My God! My God! It's really you!'

'Hello,' I said, surprised that I couldn't remember her name. Her hair was in the same blonde bob, and the skin around her eyes was only slightly lined. She was drunk. 'What happened to you?' she shouted above the party noise. 'You just disappeared. One day you were there, one day you weren't.'

I could feel Michael looking at me. 'I changed schools,' I said.

She clutched at my arm. 'You know Christine Quinn?

Well, of course, we all picked on you – my God, we were terrible!' She shook her head and giggled. 'Well, apparently she's in rehab, and Lucy Bishop told me her entire septum has been eaten away.' She pointed at her nose. 'That's this bit here. Can you believe it? Someone else, who was it, Eleanor I think – well, she's pregnant, apparently – said Christine tried to kill herself. They're saying overdose, but it was intentional. Heroin!' My former schoolmate checked herself. 'Or was it cocaine? Anyway, she's a mess. Can you believe it?' she cried again, and before I had to answer, another girl, one I did not recognise, leapt on her from behind and they disappeared into the smoke in an orgy of air-kissing and shrieking laughter.

So I always thought that whatever had truly happened to Christine, she'd had her comeuppance; karma had caught her and slung her into a torment of drug addiction and regret. But here she was, *here she was*, living in my neighbourhood, pregnant, attending active birth yoga classes, getting on with her life, like me.

Yesterday Paula phoned. 'Is everything all right? Why haven't you come to class?'

'Work,' I said. 'I know, I'm sorry, I've really wanted to come, but . . .'

'Well, you did pay for all of June. It seems a pity. I was worried something had happened.'

'No. No. Sorry. I'll try to make it this week.'

'Great. I could always find someone else for your place, if you don't want to continue.'

'No, I do. Sorry. I'll see you on Thursday.'

'Good.'

Aside from Christine, I am the most recent member of the class, though more pregnant than some of the other women. If you can be more or less pregnant. Further along. One day I will be the most pregnant and then it will be time to have the baby. I wonder how many weeks Christine is. That morning she came in, I cleared out of the room when all the other women still lay on the yoga mats, oblivious, perfumed lavender-bags pressed to their blinded eyes.

Michael and I made love last night, something we do rarely now that I am so big. It was intense, and sweet. Afterwards, he was dressing to go into the hospital, and I stopped in the middle of reaching down the back of the bed for the rhomboid-shaped pillow that helps support my stomach while I sleep. A question had been pressing in on my mind for days. 'What if our child is bullied at school?' I asked him, and before I could stop myself I had burst into tears.

'Hey,' he said. 'Hey.' He came and stood by me, his shirt unbuttoned and his belt undone. 'Baby. Is this something I should know about?'

It was twenty-four hours a day, five days a week, sometimes seven. It was like a constant electric drilling inside your head. Christine began to make phone-calls in the middle of the night. I begged my parents for a telephone in my room so they wouldn't find out what was going on. We sat there in the dark, on either end of the telephone wires, and she whispered at me: *We're going to do you, we're going to burn you, I'll get my cigarette and burn your face with it, my boyfriend's going to rape you, he'll rape you with a beer bottle so he doesn't have to touch your stinking cunt, if you tell anyone you're fucking dead*. The world reduced to the size of a small, dark hole. I felt like a small, dark hole, like the abortion they said I was.

It was my failing marks, in the end, that persuaded my parents I should change schools. They asked me if I agreed and I remember just nodding, mute, almost unbelieving that the life I was living might come to an end. At the same time my father got another transfer, and the easiest thing was to move once more. On my first day at the new school, Eloise told me she liked my hair and asked if I wanted to do scene painting for the mid-term play. My fidgeting and twitching impulses disappeared; my whole world expanded. I thought I was rid of Christine for ever.

The phone rang early this morning, waking me up, but it was only Michael telling me he'd be late back from his shift. 'They want me to sleep a bit here and stay on,' he said while I gripped the receiver hard, the pulse in my throat still pumping. 'But I told them no. So I'm two hours away, three at the most.'

'I love you,' I said.

'Go back to sleep,' he told me, 'and I'll come and wake you up.'

But I couldn't slip back into my dreams. The night's darkness was ebbing from the room. I got up, showered and went downstairs. Yesterday's dishes were still in the sink: Michael's strange implements, his lemon zester and his cone-shaped colander. Sometimes I wonder if he is a frustrated surgeon, but he maintains that it's making the correct diagnosis he finds the most fulfilling. The baby was very active, and I lay on the sofa to enjoy the secret turning feelings inside me. Before long the living-room curtains were glowing with pale, gauzy light, and I thought it must be time for Michael to come home. I imagined him tired, driving, needing a shave, hungry. So I came out here, to the café, to buy some pain au chocolat and plain croissants for his breakfast.

The man behind the counter wears a clean white-and blue-striped apron, and see-through plastic gloves. Baskets filled with crispy, flaky pastries, dusted just so with icing sugar, and jars of jewel-like berry preserves line the bench.

The sunlight that falls in great golden lozenges through the streak-free windows seems to carry some of the greenness of the nearby park. I can see a man over there cutting the lawns, and it might be just my imagination but I'm sure that as well as the cosy aromas of baking and hot coffee, there is the sharp scent in here of freshly cut grass. I am in a daze, cradling my stomach and watching, but not really seeing, the man carefully tong the pastries into a white paper bag, when the little brass bell above the street door tinkles – a sweet, innocuous sound – and another woman walks into the room.

The man wearing the stripy apron looks up at her and says, 'Are you all right? You're not going to have it in here, are you?'

When I turn and see her, framed by the doorway, the contours of her face in shadow. Christine's voice says, 'Oh. Hello.'

She moves into the café with the side-to-side, lumbering gait of the heavily pregnant. The skin on her cheeks is flushed red, and her eyes register shock. 'I thought I saw you the other morning,' she says, 'at Paula's class.'

Paula. She is already on friendly terms with her. My blood pressure is low: I have fainted before now in this pregnancy, but I hold on tight to the counter-top and clench my teeth to quell the dizziness. Christine's face has taken on the thickened, full-lipped look some women get, and sunlight catches the blonde fluff around her jaw. 'Do you live nearby?' she is saying. 'Where are you planning to have the baby?'

I give the café man the five-pound note from my pocket, and take the bag of croissants from him with a shaking hand. 'Thank you,' I say to him, and now I have to try to get past her and out of the door into the safety of the public street.

I am outside. It is too early: the road is empty. I start to

22

walk, fast, in the direction of home, but hear the café door creak and swing behind me and Christine is calling my name. And so I begin to run. It's hard with the baby and my breasts are sore. Our street appears on my right and I stumble. I can't go up there, Michael might not be back and I can't be near my home with her, I can't have her know where I live. There's a stitch in my side, and my stomach hurts with the impact of each step. She's still calling after me and it strikes me how ridiculous we must look – two enormous women running full-tilt towards the swelling hills of the park – and a weird laugh rises up in my throat but I swallow it back. I have to outpace her, I must get away.

But the muscles above my pelvis contract, everything tightens over the bump, and I reach one of the painted wooden benches and sit down, panting, my mouth dry. Christine approaches.

'I want to talk to you,' she says.

'Why?' I tell myself I'm not going to cry. I can feel in the crown of my scalp the twitch, the nodding tic, wanting to return, and I rub at the skin hard with my hand. 'There's nothing to say.'

'Please,' she says. 'I want to – I want to say I'm sorry.'

Something in me makes me look at her, although I don't believe anything she says. My breathing still comes fast and shallow. 'You'll never know what you did to me,' I say.

'I'm so sorry.' Her voice breaks. She begins to cry. 'It's haunted me, what we did, I was so unhappy but once I'd started, I couldn't stop.' Her shoulders heave up and down; she shakes her head. Her face is an open bucket of misery. 'When I saw you the other day, I knew – I knew it would all come back to get me, the way I was, the disgusting things.' She holds her belly, still crying. 'And the baby will pay, I'm sure of it. How can I be a good mother? There'll be something wrong.'

Somewhere, somewhere deep inside me, a jammed-up catch clicks, and a key turns, and a tiny pocket of held breath is released. 'How many weeks are you?' I ask.

She sniffs, juddery. 'Thirty-five. I'm sorry, I have no right to do this. I wondered for so long what happened to you and now this – it's so strange.'

I've never felt like the kind of person people wondered about after they had gone. 'I'm not sure what I can say to you,' I tell her.

'If my husband knew,' she says, 'if anybody knew . . .'

'Are you still going to the yoga class?'

'No. Haven't you been? I thought you were a regular.'

'I am,' I say. And up the path that cuts a diagonal from our street corner to this bench comes a tall, broad figure, waving at me, calling something. Michael reaches us, and I love his tired face, the purple beneath his eyes, the unkempt hair and his cigarette-stained teeth so much, I smile. 'Hi.'

'I thought it was you,' he says, and nods at Christine. 'Hello.' He looks closer – he's good at looking closer – and notices that she's been crying. 'Are you all right?'

The bomb scares are more frequent now that the weather's getting warmer. Some days, according to the news reports, the entire city grinds to a halt, but you wouldn't know it here, in the peaceful streets where we live. A kid rode past me in the park today, a teenage boy on a pushbike, wheeling along the curved pathways through the smoothly mown grass. He wore a plastic mask on his face, like a dinner plate with the eyes and mouth cut out, half of it black and half of it white. Through the mouth-hole he was trying to smoke a cigarette. This wasn't easy: the bike lurched and wobbled under his single hand, and he nearly rode into a group of younger children. He seemed very alone. I don't know what he was doing with the mask; it is ages until Halloween. We've got the whole of summer before then, I thought, feeling the soft hand of sunlight warm on my belly and my face. I lay back on the grass and rested my head on the grocery bag. It was uncomfortable, lumpy with baking ingredients, but I didn't mind. By Halloween, the baby will be over three months old.

'I wanted you to have a different life from mine,' my mother, who has worked as a receptionist for twenty-seven years, said to me not so long ago. 'It's great that you're happy with Michael, and everything.' She paused, and I braced myself for the questions about my career, and the: 'Hasn't Eloise done so well?' followed by: 'Sometimes I don't understand your choices.' But what she said in the end was, 'We all want different things, I suppose, for our babies.' In the mermaid room I want for my baby, there will be angelfish, and coral, and a barnacled chest spilling ruby-rimmed goblets, and long, long ropes of pearls.

# Love at First Sight
## *Polly Samson*

The doctor climbed the five flights to my flat, bitter with lumbago and the bloody law that demanded he climb these stairs at all. He had been summoned, despite my protestations, by the midwives. 'Sorry,' they said. 'It's an NHS rule.' They were gone now, and we were three, alone; cocooned with cushions and quilts and soft shawls. We were strange and warm and new. We were waiting for the bad fairy to appear. From the bedroom, we could hear his leather trench-coat slap-slapping against his boots as he marched nearer. Charlie was snuggled, fists closed around the curls of new lambskin, the first sleep out of the womb, perfect. The doctor pushed past my baby's father, to point a long finger at me. 'You, you're irresponsible,' he said, and I thought again how much he resembled the child-catcher in *Chitty Chitty Bang Bang*.

'You wouldn't be smiling like that if something had gone wrong,' he said. Then he snatched up my sleeping baby and sneezed in his face.

'Out,' said my boyfriend. 'Get out!'

Nine months earlier, this same doctor had the strangest reaction when I informed him that I was pregnant. He said: 'And what do you expect me to do about that?' When I replied that I just thought he should know, he looked so downcast that I found myself mumbling apologetically about world overpopulation, Chinese girls, Romanian orphans, grain-shortages, children in care.

'I see,' he said, fixing me with a disappointed eye, while I rubbed my tummy through my jeans. 'But you want to *keep* the baby?'

I stuck to the ante-natal appointments that Dr Child-snatcher arranged at the teaching hospital closest to my office – it worked out cheaper that way. But I was lying through my teeth each time I confirmed that I would indeed be having my baby there, in one of the terrifying steel beds on wheels that they showed me. These hospital beds were the stuff of my nightmares, the curtains that pulled right around, clattering like a brisk telling-off. And the all-too-obvious metaphor of the hospital corridor made me shiver too. At the end there's terror and white light, bright enough to penetrate your eyelids.

In the early stages of pregnancy, I spent my lunch-hours – and then some – waiting, waiting, at the hospital, hugging myself with the thrill of deception. I sat smirking and secretive and others smiled back sometimes, their faces pale and puffy under sick neon tubes, and nothing much to look at but the gory video-loops of beached women, screaming and bloody, their babies' heads emerging from between their legs like leaching beetroot. Later, when the routine checks became weekly, I was spared the flickering fluorescence, the blood-curdling soundtrack, and instead was back with my doctor, bringing to his surgery a sample of early-morning urine. Each week when I presented him with the jar, warm from my pocket, Dr Child-catcher would look at me over his half-moons and say: 'And what can I do for you?'

As far as he was concerned, I would be going to the hospital for the birth; that was the rule then – first babies, and all that. But I was arrogant and my boyfriend had a friend who was a charismatic French obstetrician. He told me: 'You will have your *bébé* how your mother had you.'

My mother popped me into the world at home in Crouch End in a room with a bay window to the street. One of the first things she did after the birth was to stick her maroon knitted mittens on my feet because she thought they looked cold. When the midwife finally arrived, short-of-breath and dishevelled, my mother already had me in her arms. She told the flustered woman not to fuss because for her it was nothing: 'No worse than bad constipation.'

'Well, I never,' said this midwife, who was old and, so they tell me, almost blind. I imagine her peering close, possibly through glasses mended with plasters. 'And look what she's wearing on her feet! What were you expecting, a little monkey?'

My mother prided herself on providing a positive image of birth. She's the sort of woman that Gauguin might have painted. Strong and dark, she looks like a woman who would squat down in the field, have her baby, and continue on her way. 'And when I held you,' she said, 'the waves of love were more powerful than any pain.'

It will be love at first sight. It *will* be love at first sight. That's what they tell you. They tell you about deep eye-contact. It will be impossible to look away, they say.

My firstborn lay, bubbling with mucus, tummy-down on the bedroom carpet. The charming French obstetrician, having stayed on my sofa throughout two nights of 'pre-labour', had missed the baby's arrival by a few hours, his toothbrush packed away smartish into a natty little overnight case.

'You will have to go to the hospital,' he said, having informed us, most plausibly, that he would miss his flight to Italy if he stayed for even one more contraction. 'The hospital is not so bad,' he said.

But it was too late for all that: he had already told me how unsuitable hospitals were as places for birth, how *interventionist* every consultant, how full of germs for the new *bébé* it would all be. One look at my face must have convinced him that he ought to pull an alternative out of the hat.

'I know a girl,' he said, suddenly inspired as his check-in time grew closer. 'Her name is Katie,' and he gave me her phone number as he flew out of the door. He was probably already speaking at his conference in Milan as my baby drew his first breaths.

'I wonder if it's a girl or a boy?' said Katie, the more glamorous of the two midwives who, at remarkably short notice, had supported my weight, on chairs, one either side, while I crouched and pushed and shouted that I'd changed my mind; Katie and Martha now had scratches on their thighs to prove it.

'Let's see, shall we?' said Katie brightly.

I was lost in thinking about my boyfriend, about how loud I had just screamed as the baby's head was born. It felt searing, like a Chinese burn, only hotter. My boyfriend was in the next room, as agreed, but the walls were thin. Katie was prompting me to take my baby into my arms, to have a look, but I was too shocked; in fact, I had started to shake all over and I thought I might be about to cry.

'I wonder, is it a boy or a girl?' she tried prompting me again.

'Bit hard to tell, really,' replied Martha, looking down at the baby, still lying tummy to the floor, and giving me a nudge.

'Boy or girl, bit hard to tell,' Katie repeated. The bedroom door flew open. My boyfriend stood there, crackling with dread.

'My God, please, no!' he cried, staring at the snuffling baby at my feet. 'Please, not a hermaphrodite!'

29

I was trembling and laughing, but still all I could think was: I hope my boyfriend likes this baby.

This baby was a shocker: astonishingly long, with the muscular back of an athlete. I had been expecting a mouse-sized child, a bit floppier somehow. The size of my bulge had not prepared me for a whopper: he must have been tightly packed, like a Jack in the Box. Katie measured him twice. He stretched a full twenty-four inches away from me, from the purple backs of his heels to the cap of his head which had been squeezed into the shape of a parking cone.

'A boy,' breathed his father when, finally, I brought him into my arms. My boyfriend had two daughters already, now he had a son. Had I done well? Did he love our baby? It seemed too pathetic to ask, but I was consumed with needing to know.

'Will you look at that,' said my boyfriend, grinning, crying. 'His scrotum's bigger than mine!'

Guiltily, I held my baby closer. I hadn't imagined that he'd weigh anything, that he'd feel this solid. I was waiting for something to happen. 'He looks just like you,' someone said. 'He looks like you both.' He hadn't cried yet, but Katie said it didn't matter. I thought of Narcissus and his pond. I looked down and caught his eye. It was a bright black marble, unblinking and so penetrating that it was like staring at the sun and I had to look away.

It's a decade later. We're in an ambulance and I'm watching Charlie's eyes, praying; praying to a God that my atheist parents assured me did not exist. Charlie's pupils dilate as oxygen flows from the mask. I am assailed by a memory of my grandmother. She's pale as wax, she's laying her hand on her son's coffin. 'No one should have to outlive their child,' she says. Love at first sight is mere romance compared to this.

When they loaded him on to the stretcher, after the emergency doctor – the too-young, too-pretty, hopeless, emergency doctor – had wrung her hands, unable to tell me why he couldn't breathe, refusing to tell me that he would live, he stared at me with the same intensity as the day he was born.

The ambulance man smiles at me. We talk about Harry Potter because the new one's due out tomorrow. I think: Please God, don't let him die before he's read it. I say: 'You'll be fine now,' and it's hard not to look away because I don't want him to see the doubt in my eyes.

On the day he was born, the Berlin Wall was breached. There was a big black headline on the front of the *Evening Standard*: GREAT DAY FOR FREEDOM, CHARLIE COMES DOWN. I'm boasting, ecstatic. Had the Wall remained, I explain, he would have been Moby, because that was top of our name-list, not Charlie, so, if only for that, he should be thankful for the collapse of Communism.

Before I started gabbling, the registrar at the hospital had wanted to write his name as *Charles*. Charlie, with the kindly air of talking to an imbecile to which mothers of ten-year-old boys must become accustomed, tells me it's time to calm down. It's possible to laugh now that he's been nebulised and stabilised. In fact, my husband, David, and I are verging on hysteria. Everything's suddenly so funny – the fact that the ambulance wouldn't start, that the emergency doctor didn't recognise a case of (alarming rather than life-threatening) croup when she saw it. Charlie points to the Zed Bed set up next to his hospital bed. 'Could we get a double?' he asks. 'There's no way my mum and dad will both fit in there,' and we collapse, giggling, on to it.

As I lie in the dark, too rich in adrenalin for sleep (in any case they're still checking Charlie's blood pressure every hour), I think how I have slept in hospital with both of my younger sons – each on their day of birth, but only once on purpose – but never before with Charlie. I can hear a baby crying, inconsolably it seems, further down the corridor.

Charlie, awake again, turns his head on the pillow and, whispering, asks me whether I really would have been so cruel as to name him Moby. 'It was either that, or Fin,' I say, biting my lips, trying to contain my mirth. I tell him how his father and I didn't know that he would be a boy until he was born. When they did the scan and we tried to see, not wanting to see, but trying all the same, joking and high at the first sighting of our baby, the scan-operator snapped: 'We're not here to make pretty pictures for you, you know.' I tell Charlie what his name would have been, had he been a girl. 'Ugh,' he says, and I remember my Cousin Melissa having much the same reaction. 'Ugh, not *Delphi*,' she said. 'Sounds like a feminine deodorant.'

It was different with David, when our first baby together was scanned. Things had moved on, ante-natal care seemed kinder somehow. Maybe it was just because it was a different hospital and Dr Child-catcher was nothing but a bad memory. Maybe it was because Charlie's father and I had something about us that shrieked 'irresponsible', like a bubble over our heads announcing that we'd break apart before our son's first birthday. Maybe everyone could see this bubble – Dr Child-catcher, the scan-nurse in the hospital, the woman who looked at me with sad eyes in Mothercare – who knows?

As David and I marvelled at the sight of our twenty-week-old foetus waving at us through a snowstorm, Bill, the scan-man, asked if we would like to know the sex. 'Yes,' said David. 'No,' said I. We decided that Bill would write it on a piece of paper to allow time for democracy.

We could always destroy the paper if David could be persuaded not to cheat fate. Of course, the moment I hopped out of the car to buy milk on the way home, David peeked, and the moment I returned, I could tell that he had, the sneak.

'Sonny' – that's what Charlie wanted to call the little boy that everyone now knew we were having. I remember him, jaw set with grim determination, as he said: 'If you won't call the baby "Sonny" he'll have to be "Dead Salmon".' At five years old the apple of my eye was finding it hard to adjust to the idea of a little brother.

'Come in and meet baby Joe,' we said when Charlie arrived at the hospital, clutching a fruit cake which had *Congratulations* piped on the top in icing. Joe was a little sleeping Buddha at my side. I hoped that the tubes that stretched from my arms to the drip wouldn't give Charlie a fright. They looked like red liquorice bootlaces. I had to lie still and could only look at Joe from the corner of my eye.

'Hello, little baby Dead Salmon,' said Charlie.

Joe had been born the night before, at home, and with such ease that Charlie, asleep upstairs, had not been woken. Until the sudden medical emergency, my concerns were that my new baby was rather fat and pink. 'Do you think he's lovely?' I whispered. 'Are you pleased?' With echoes of Charlie's birth, I was waiting for my husband's rapture before I was free to focus on the love that I had once again failed to deliver at first sight. As it turned out, that was the least of my problems that night.

'You have a heart-shaped womb,' the consultant had told me when I came round from the anaesthetic on a hospital trolley.

'Thank you,' I said, because there's something about being told that you have a heart-shaped womb that makes it seem like a compliment. How romantic! Better than a kidney-shaped womb, or an ordinary round one, like a balloon.

'That's why the placenta got stuck,' he said, and he explained that I'd lost almost five pints of blood before I'd reached the hospital.

I remembered him from the night before, from when they wheeled me into the operating theatre; new baby Joe somewhere else, not with me. The consultant's face was looming and blurred then, close to mine then far, far away, masked, only his eyes showing.

'Tell me I won't die,' I had said, and his reply was: 'I'm not God.'

'Remember, there is no God.' My grandmother often told me about coming to see me on the day I was born. My brothers were there, leaning over the carry-cot, repeating the mantra: 'Now, Polly, remember, there is no God.' It was this mantra, my brothers' boyhood voices, that I heard as I sank into anaesthesia.

My brothers were already my mother's sons for six and seven years before she met my father, but I was my father's first child. I hated being a one-off. More than once I begged my mother for a younger sibling but she always said: 'After you?' Or: 'One like you is enough, thank you.' Or: 'Not bloody likely!' And my dad just chuckled but I didn't get the joke. I suppose I thought that if the recipe were any good, it'd be worth repeating.

In bed, forty or so weeks before my third baby was born, my husband said to me (at the crucial, sacred, stay-or-go moment), 'So what. We make lovely babies.' The earth moved. And then, so did the emergency services. The fire brigade this time. Quite what they were doing bursting into our hotel room at midnight we never did find out. But I didn't have a care. I was loved enough.

'So what,' he said. 'We make lovely babies.' My third baby lay in my arms. I breathed him in. The top of his head was for nuzzling, so warm and buttery. His pastel face was smooth and sweet as a sugared almond. He was newborn Charlie and newborn Joe, and he was newborn himself. I wouldn't have been able to tear my eyes away from his even if I had wanted to. It was only later, as he slept moulded to my belly, that I realised that I hadn't counted his fingers and toes, or looked for faults, or wasted time wondering if his father liked him: love is like that.

# A Letter To Our Son

## *Peter Carey*

Before I have finished writing this, the story of how you were born, I will be forty-four years old and the events and feelings which make up the story will be at least eight months old. You are lying in the next room in a cotton jump-suit. You have five teeth. You cannot walk. You do not seem interested in crawling. You are sound asleep.

I have put off writing this so long that, now the time is here, I do not want to write it. I cannot think. Laziness. Wooden shutters over the memory. Nothing comes, no pictures, no feelings, but the architecture of the hospital at Camperdown.

You were born in the King George V Hospital in Missenden Road, Camperdown, a building that won an award for its architecture. It was opened during the Second World War, but its post-Bauhaus modern style has its roots in that time before the First World War, with an optimism about the technological future that we may never have again.

I liked this building. I liked its smooth, rounded, shiny corners. I liked its wide stairs, I liked the huge sash-windows, even the big blue-and-white checked tiles: when I remember this building there is sunshine splashed across those tiles, but there were times when it seemed that other memories might triumph and it would be remembered for the harshness of its neon lights and emptiness of the corridors.

A week before you were born, I sat with your mother in a four-bed ward on the eleventh floor of this building. In this ward she received blood transfusions from plum-red plastic bags suspended on rickety stainless-steel stands. The blood did not always flow smoothly. The bags had to be fiddled with, the stand had to be raised, lowered, have its drip-rate increased, decreased, inspected by the sister who had been a political prisoner in Chile, by the sister from the Solomon Islands, by others I don't remember. The blood entered your mother through a needle in her forearm. When the vein collapsed, a new one had to be found. This was caused by a kind of bruising called 'tissuing'. We soon knew all about tissuing. It made her arm hurt like hell.

She was bright-eyed and animated as always, but her lips had a slight blue tinge and her skin had a tight, translucent quality.

She was in this room on the west because her blood appeared to be dying. Some thought the blood was killing itself. This is what we all feared, none more than me, for when I heard her blood-count was so low, the first thing I thought (stop that thought, cut it off, bury it) was cancer.

This did not necessarily have a lot to do with Alison, but with me, and how I had grown up, with a mother who was preoccupied with cancer and who, going into surgery for suspected breast cancer, begged the doctor to 'cut them both off'. When my mother's friend Enid Tanner boasted of her hard stomach muscles, my mother envisaged a growth. When her father complained of a sore elbow, my mother threatened the old man: 'All right, we'll take you up to Doctor Campbell and she'll cut it off.' When I was ten, my mother's brother got cancer and they cut his leg off right up near the hip and took photographs of him, naked, one-legged, to show other doctors the success of the operation.

When I heard your mother's blood-count was low, I was my mother's son. I thought: cancer.

I remembered what Alison had told me of that great tragedy of her grandparents' life, how their son (her uncle) had leukaemia, how her grandfather then bought him the car (a Ford Prefect? a Morris Minor?) he had hitherto refused him, how the dying boy had driven for miles and miles, hours and hours while his cells attacked each other.

I tried to stop this thought, to cut it off. It grew again, like a thistle whose root has not been removed and must grow again, every time, stronger and stronger.

The best haematological unit in Australia was on hand to deal with the problem. They worked in the hospital across the road, the Royal Prince Alfred. They were friendly and efficient. They were not at all like I had imagined big hospital specialists to be. They took blood samples, but the blood did not tell them enough. They returned to take marrow from your mother's bones. They brought a big needle with them that would give you the horrors if you could see the size of it.

The doctor's speciality was leukaemia, but he said to us: 'We don't think it's anything really nasty.' Thus 'nasty' became a code for cancer.

They diagnosed megaloblastic anaemia which, although we did not realise it, is the condition of the blood and not the disease itself.

Walking back through the streets in Shimbashi in Tokyo, your mother once told me that a fortune-teller had told her she would die young. It was for this reason – or so I remembered – that she took such care of her health. At the time she told me this, we had not known each other very long. It was July. We had fallen in love in May. We were still stumbling over each other's feelings in the dark. I took this secret of your mother's lightly, not thinking about the weight it must carry, what it might mean to talk about it. I hurt her; we fought, in the street by the Shimbashi railway station, in a street with shop windows advertising cosmetic surgery, in the Dai-Ichi Hotel in the Ginza district of Tokyo, Japan.

When they took the bone marrow from your mother's spine, I held her hand. The needle had a cruel diameter, was less a needle than an instrument for removing a plug. She was very brave. Her wrists seemed too thin, her skin too white and shiny, her eyes too big and bright. She held my hand because of pain. I held hers because I loved her, because I could not think of living if I did not have her. I thought of what she had told me in Tokyo. I wished there was a God I could pray to.

I flew to Canberra on 7 May 1984. It was my forty-first birthday. I had injured my back and should have been lying flat on a board. I had come from a life with a woman which had reached, for both of us, a state of chronic unhappiness. I will tell you the truth: I was on that aeroplane to Canberra because I hoped I might fall in love. This made me a dangerous person.

There was a playwrights' conference in Canberra. I hoped there would be a woman there who would love me as I would love her. This was a fantasy I had had before, getting on aeroplanes to foreign cities, riding in taxis towards hotels in Melbourne, in Adelaide, in Brisbane. I do not mean that I was thinking about sex, or an affair, but that I was looking for someone to spend my life with. Also – and I swear I have not invented this after the fact – I had a vision of your mother's neck.

I hardly knew her. I met her once at a dinner when I scarcely noticed her. I met her a second time when I saw, in a meeting room, the back of her neck. We spoke that time, but I was argumentative and I did not think of her in what I can only call 'that way'.

And yet as the aeroplane came down to land in Canberra, I saw your mother's neck, and thought: Maybe Alison Summers will be there. She was the dramaturge at the Nimrod Theatre. It was a playwrights' conference. She should be there.

And she was. And we fell in love. And we stayed up till four in the morning every morning talking. And there were other men, everywhere, in love with her. I didn't know about the other men. I knew only that I was in love as I had not been since I was eighteen years old. I wanted to marry Alison Summers, and at the end of the first night we had been out together, when I walked her to the door of her room, and we had, for the first time, ever so lightly, kissed on the lips – and also, I must tell you, for it was delectable and wonderful, I kissed your mother on her long, beautiful neck – and when we had kissed and patted the air between us and said, 'All right,' a number of times, and I had walked back to my room where I had, because of my back injury, a thin mattress lying flat on the floor, and when I was in this bed, I said, aloud, to the empty room: 'I am going to live with Alison.'

And I went to sleep so happy I must have been smiling.

She did not know what I told the room. And it was three or four days before I could see her again, three or four days before we could go out together, spend time alone, and I could tell her what I thought.

I had come to Canberra wanting to fall in love. Now I was in love. Who was I in love with? I hardly knew, and yet I knew exactly. I did not even realise how beautiful she was. I found that out later. At the beginning I recognised something more potent than beauty: it was a force, a life, an energy. She had such life in her face, in her eyes – those eyes which you inherited – most of all. It was this I loved, this which I recognised so that I could say – having kissed her so lightly – *I will live with Alison*. And know that I was right.

It was a conference. We were behaving like men and women do at conferences, having affairs. We would not be so sleazy. After four nights staying up talking till four a.m. we had still not made love. I would creep back to my room, to my mattress on the floor. We talked about everything. Your mother liked me, but I cannot tell you how long it took her to fall in love with me. But I know we were discussing marriage and babies when we had not even been to bed together. That came early one morning when I returned to her room after three hours' sleep. We had not planned to make love there at the conference but there we were, lying on the bed, kissing, and then we were making love, and you were not conceived then, of course, and yet from that time we never ceased thinking of you and when, later in Sydney, we had to learn to adjust to each other's needs, and when we argued, which we did often then, it was you more than anything that kept us together. We wanted you so badly. We loved you before we saw you. We loved you as we made you, in bed in another room, at Lovett Bay.

When your mother came to the eleventh floor of the King George V Hospital, you were almost ready to be born. Every day the sisters came and smeared jelly on your mother's tight, bulging stomach and then stuck a flat little octopus-type sucker to it and listened to the noises you made.

You sounded like soldiers marching on a bridge.

You sounded like short-wave radio.

You sounded like the inside of the sea.

We did not know if you were a boy or a girl, but we called you Sam anyway. When you kicked or turned we said, 'Sam's doing his exercises.' We said silly things.

When we heard how low Alison's blood-count was, I phoned the obstetrician to see if you were OK. She said there was no need to worry. She said you had your own blood-supply. She said that as long as the mother's count was above six there was no need to worry.

Your mother's count was 6.2. This was very close. I kept worrying that you had been hurt in some way. I could not share this worry, for to share it would only be to make it worse. Also, I recognise that I have made a whole career out of making my anxieties get up and walk around, not only in my own mind, but in the minds of readers. I went to see a naturopath once. We talked about negative emotions – fear and anger. I said to him, 'But I *use* my anger and my fear.' I talked about these emotions as if they were chisels and hammers.

This alarmed him considerably.

Your mother is not like this. When the haematologists saw how she looked, they said: 'Our feeling is that you don't have anything nasty.' They topped her up with blood until her count was twelve and although they had not located the source of her anaemia, they sent her home.

A few days later her count was down to just over six.

It seemed as if there was a silent civil war inside her veins and arteries. The number of casualties was appalling.

I think we both got frightened then. I remember coming home to Louisa Road. I remember worrying that I would cry. I remember embracing your mother – and you too, for you were a great bulge between us. I must not cry. I must support her.

I made a meal. It was salade niçoise. The electric lights, in memory, were all ten watts, sapped by misery. I could barely eat. I think we may have watched a funny film on videotape. We repacked the bag that had been unpacked so short a time before. It now seemed likely that your birth was to be induced. If your mother was sick she could not be looked after properly with you inside her. She would be given one more blood transfusion, and then the induction would begin. And that is how your birthday would be on September the thirteenth.

Two nights before your birthday I sat with Alison in the four-bed ward, the one facing east, towards Missenden Road. The curtains were drawn around us. I sat on the bed and held her hand. The blood continued its slow viscous drip from the plum-red bag along the clear plastic tube and into her arm. The obstetrician was with us. She stood at the head of the bed, a kind, intelligent woman in her early thirties. We talked about Alison's blood. We asked her what she thought this mystery could be. Really what we wanted was to be told that everything was OK. There was a look on Alison's face when she asked. I cannot describe it, but it was not a face seeking medical 'facts'.

The obstetrician went through all the things that were not wrong with your mother's blood. She did not have a vitamin B deficiency. She did not have a folic acid deficiency. There was no iron deficiency. She did not have any of the common (and easily fixable) anaemias of pregnancy. So what could it be, we asked, really only wishing to be assured it was nothing 'nasty'.

'Well,' said the obstetrician, 'at this stage you cannot rule out cancer.'

I watched your mother's face. Nothing in her expression showed what she must feel. There was a slight colouring of her cheeks. She nodded. She asked a question or two. She held my hand, but there was no tight squeezing.

The obstetrician asked Alison if she was going to be 'all right'. Alison said she would be 'all right'. But when the obstetrician left she left the curtains drawn.

The obstetrician's statement was not of course categorical, and not everyone who has cancer dies, but Alison was, at that instant, confronting the thing that we fear most. When the doctor said those words, it was like a dream or a nightmare. I heard them said. And yet they were not said. They could not be said. And when we hugged each other – when the doctor had gone – we pressed our bodies together as we always had before, and if there were tears on our cheeks, there had been tears on our cheeks before. I kissed your mother's eyes. Her hair was wet with her tears. I smoothed her hair on her forehead. My own eyes were swimming. She said: 'All right, how are we going to get through all this?'

Now you know her, you know how much like her that is. She is not going to be a victim of anything.

'We'll decide it's going to be OK,' she said, 'that's all.'

And we dried our eyes.

But that night, when she was alone in her bed, waiting for the sleeping pill to work, she thought: If I die, I'll at least have made this little baby.

When I left your mother I appeared dry-eyed and positive, but my disguise was a frail shell of a thing and it cracked on the stairs and my grief and rage came spilling out in gulps. The halls of the hospital gleamed with polish and vinyl and fluorescent light. The flower-seller on the ground floor had locked up his shop. The foyer was empty. The whisker-shadowed man in Admissions was watching television. In Missenden Road two boys in jeans and sandshoes conducted separate conversations in separate phone booths. Death was not touching them. They turned their backs to each other. One of them – a red-head with a tattoo on his forearm – laughed.

In Missenden Road there were taxis NOT FOR HIRE speeding towards other destinations.

In Missenden Road the bright white lights above the zebra crossings became a luminous sea inside my eyes. Car lights turned into necklaces and ribbons. I was crying, thinking: It is not for me to cry. Crying is a poison, a negative force; everything will be all right – but I was weeping as if huge balloons of air had to be released from inside my guts. I walked normally. My grief was invisible. A man rushed past me, carrying roses wrapped in cellophane. I got into my car. The floor was littered with car-park tickets from all the previous days of blood transfusions, tests, test results, admission etc. I drove out of the car park. I talked aloud.

I told the night I loved Alison Summers. I love you, I love you, you will not die. There were red lights at the Parramatta Road. I sat there, howling, unroadworthy. I love you.

The day after tomorrow there will be a baby. Will the baby have a mother? What would we do if we knew Alison was dying? What would we do so Sam would know his mother? Would we make a videotape? Would we hire a camera? Would we set it up and act for you? Would we talk to you with smiling faces, showing you how we were together, how we loved each other? How could we? How could we think of these things?

I was a prisoner in a nightmare driving down Ross Street in Glebe. I passed the Afrikan restaurant where your mother and I ate after first coming to live in Balmain.

All my life I have waited for this woman. This cannot happen.

I thought: Why would it *not* happen? Every day people are tortured, killed, bombed. Every day babies starve. Every day there is pain and grief, enough to make you howl to the moon for ever. Why should we be exempt, I thought, from the pain of life?

What would I do with a baby? How would I look after

it? Day after day, minute after minute, by myself. I would be a sad man, forever marked by the loss of this woman. I would love the baby. I would care for it. I would see, in its features, every day, the face of the woman I had loved more than any other.

When I think of this time, it seems as if it's two in the morning, but it was not. It was ten o'clock at night. I drove home through a landscape of grotesque imaginings.

The house was empty and echoing.

In the nursery everything was waiting for you, all the things we had got for 'the baby'. We had read so many books about babies, been to classes where we learned about how babies are born, but we still did not understand the purpose of all the little clothes we had folded in the drawers. We did not know which was a swaddle and which was a sheet. We could not have selected the clothes to dress you in.

I drank coffee. I drank wine. I set out to telephone Kathy Lette, Alison's best friend, so she would have this 'news' before she spoke to your mother the next day. I say 'set out' because each time I began to dial, I thought: I am not going to do this properly. I hung up. I did deep breathing. I calmed myself. I telephoned. Kim Williams, Kathy's husband, answered and said Kathy was not home yet. I thought: She must know. I told Kim, and as I told him the weeping came with it. I could hear myself. I could imagine Kim listening to me. I would sound frightening, grotesque, and less in control than I was. When I had finished frightening him, I went to bed and slept.

I do not remember the next day, only that we were bright and determined. Kathy hugged Alison and wept. I hugged Kathy and wept. There were isolated incidents. We were 'handling it'. And, besides, you were coming on the next day. You were life, getting stronger and stronger.

I had practical things to worry about. For instance: the bag. The bag was to hold all the things for the labour ward. There was a list for the contents of the bag and these contents were all purchased and ready, but still I must bring them to the hospital early the next morning. I checked the bag. I placed things where I would not forget them. You wouldn't believe the things we had. We had a cassette-player and a tape with soothing music. We had rosemary and lavender oil so I could massage your mother and relax her between contractions. I had a Thermos to fill with blocks of frozen orange juice. There were special cold packs to relieve the pain of a backache labour. There were paper pants – your arrival, after all, was not to happen without a great deal of mess. There were socks, because your mother's feet would almost certainly get very cold. I packed all these things, and there was something in the process of this packing which helped overcome my fears and made me concentrate on you, our little baby, already so loved although we did not know your face, had seen no more of you than the ghostly blue image thrown up by the ultrasound in the midst of whose shifting perspectives we had seen your little hand move. ('He waved to us.')

On the morning of the day of your birth I woke early. It was only just light. I had notes stuck on the fridge and laid out on the table. I made coffee and poured it into a Thermos. I made the bagel sandwiches your mother and I had planned months before – my lunch. I filled the bagels with a fiery Polish sausage and cheese and gherkins. For your mother, I filled a spray-bottle with Evian water.

It was a Saturday morning and bright and sunny and I knew you would be born but I did not know what it would be like. I drove along Ross Street in Glebe ignorant of the important things I would know that night. I wore grey stretchy trousers and a black shirt which would later be marked by the white juices of your birth. I was excited, but less than you might imagine. I parked at the hospital as I had parked on all those other occasions. I carried the bags up to the eleventh floor. They were heavy.

Alison was in her bed. She looked calm and beautiful. When we kissed, her lips were soft and tender. She said: 'This time tomorrow we'll have a little baby.'

In our conversation, we used the diminutive a lot. You were always spoken of as 'little', as indeed you must really have been, but we would say 'little' hand, 'little' feet, 'little' baby, and thus evoked all our powerful feelings about you.

This term ('little') is so loaded that writers are wary of using it. It is cute, sentimental, 'easy'. All of sentient life seems programmed to respond to 'little'. If you watch grown dogs with a pup, a pup they have never seen, they are immediately patient and gentle, even solicitous, with it. If you had watched your mother and father holding up a tiny terry-towelling jump-suit in a department store, you would have seen their faces change as they celebrated your 'littleness' while, at the same time, making fun of their own responses – they were aware of acting in a way they would have previously thought of as saccharine.

And yet we were not aware of the torrents of emotion your 'littleness' would unleash in us, and by the end of September the thirteenth we would think it was nothing other than the meaning of life itself.

When I arrived at the hospital with the heavy bags of cassette-players and rosemary oil, I saw a dark-bearded, neat man in a suit sitting out by the landing. This was the hypnotherapist who had arrived to help you come into the world. He was serious, impatient, eager to start. He wanted to start in the pathology ward, but in the end he helped carry the cassette-player, Thermoses, sandwiches, massage oil, sponges, paper pants, apple juice, frozen orange blocks, rolling pin, cold packs, and even water down to the labour ward where – on a stainless-steel stand eight feet high – the sisters were already hanging the bag of Oxytocin which would ensure this day was your birthday.

It was a pretty room, by the taste of the time. As I write it is still that time, and I still think it pretty. All the surfaces were hospital surfaces – easy to clean – laminexes, vinyls, materials with a hard shininess, but with colours that were soft pinks and blues and an effect that was unexpectedly pleasant, even sophisticated.

The bed was one of those complicated stainless-steel machines which seem so cold and impersonal until you realise all the clever things they can do. In the wall there were sockets with labels like 'Oxygen'. The cupboards were filled with paper-wrapped sterile 'objects'. There was, in short, a seriousness about the room, and when we plugged in the cassette-player we took care to make sure we were not using a socket that might be required for something more important.

The hypnotherapist left me to handle the unpacking of the bags. He explained his business to the obstetrician. She told him that eight hours would be a good, fast labour. The hypnotherapist said he and Alison were aiming for three. I don't know what the doctor thought, but I thought there was not a hope in hell.

When the Oxytocin drip had been put into my darling's arm, when the water-clear hormone was entering her veins, one drip every ten seconds (you could hear the machine click when a drip was released), when these pure chemical messages were being delivered to her body, the hypnotherapist attempted to send other messages of a less easily assayable quality.

I tell you the truth: I did not care for this hypnotherapist, this pushy, over-eager fellow taking up all this room in the labour ward. He sat on the right-hand side of the bed. I sat on the left. He made me feel useless. He said: 'You are going to have a good labour, a fast labour, a fast labour like the one you have already visualised.' Your mother's eyes were closed. She had such large, soft lids, such tender and vulnerable coverings of skin. Inside the pink light of the womb, your eyelids were the same. Did you hear the messages your mother was sending to her body and to you? The hypnotherapist said: 'After just three hours you are going to deliver a baby, a good, strong, healthy baby. It will be an easy birth, an effortless birth. It will last three hours and you will not tear.' On the door the sisters had tacked a sign reading: QUIET PLEASE. HYPNOTHERAPY IN PROGRESS. 'You are going to be so relaxed, and in a moment you are going to be even more relaxed, more relaxed than you have ever been before. You are feeling yourself going deeper and deeper, and when you come to, you will be in a state of waking hypnosis and you will respond to the trigger-words Peter will give you during your labour, words which will make you, once again, so relaxed.'

My trigger-words were to be 'Breathe' and 'Relax'.

The hypnotherapist gave me his phone number and asked me to call when you were born. But for the moment you had not felt the effects of the Oxytocin on your world and you could not yet have suspected the adventures the day would have in store for you.

You still sounded like the ocean, like soldiers marching across a bridge, like short-wave radio.

On Tuesday nights through the previous winter we had gone to classes in a building where the lifts were always sticking. We had walked up the stairs to a room where pregnant women and their partners had rehearsed birth with dolls, had watched hours of videotapes of exhausted women in labour. We had practised all the different sorts of breathing. We had learned of the different positions for giving birth: the squat, the supported squat, the squat supported by a seated partner. We knew the positions for first and second stage, for a backache labour, and so on, and so on. We learned birth was a complicated, exhausting and difficult process. We worried we would forget how to breathe. And yet now the time was here we both felt confident, even though nothing would be like it had been in the birth classes. Your mother was connected to the Oxytocin drip which meant she could not get up and walk around. It meant it was difficult for her to 'belly dance' or do most of the things we had spent so many evenings learning about.

In the classes they tell you that the contractions will start far apart, that you should go to hospital only when they are ten minutes apart: short bursts of pain, but long rests in between. During this period your mother could expect to walk around, to listen to music, to enjoy a massage. However, your birth was not to be like this. This was not because of you. It was because of the Oxytocin. It had a fast, intense effect, like a double Scotch when you're expecting a beer. There were not to be any ten-minute rests, and from the time the labour started it was, almost immediately, fast and furious, with a one-minute contraction followed by no more than two minutes of rest.

If there had been time to be frightened, I think I would have been frightened. Your mother was in the grip of pains she could not escape from. She squatted on a bean bag. It was as if her insides were all tangled, and tugged in a battle to the death. Blood ran from her. Fluid like egg-white. I did not know what anything was. I was a man who had wandered on to a battlefield. The blood was bright with oxygen. I wiped your mother's brow. She panted. *Huh-*

*huh-huh-huh*. I ministered to her with sponge and water. I could not take her pain for her. I could do nothing but measure the duration of the pain. I had a little red stop-watch you will one day find abandoned in a dusty drawer. (Later your mother asked me what I had felt during labour. I thought only: I must count the seconds of the contraction; I must help Alison breathe, now, now, now; I must get that sponge – there is time to make the water in the sponge cool – now I can remove that bowl and cover it. Perhaps I can reach the bottle of Evian water. God, I'm so *thirsty*. What did I think during the labour? I thought: When this contraction is over I will get to that Evian bottle.)

Somewhere in the middle of this, in these three hours in this room whose only view was a blank screen of frosted glass, I helped your mother climb on to the bed. She was on all fours. In this position she could reach the gas mask. It was nitrous oxide, laughing gas. It did not stop the pain, but it made it less important. For the gas to work your mother had to anticipate the contraction, breathing in gas before it arrived. The sister came and showed me how I could feel the contraction coming with my hand. But I couldn't. We used the stop-watch, but the contractions were not regularly spaced, and sometimes we anticipated them and sometimes not. When we did not get it right, your mother took the full brunt of the pain. She had her face close to the mattress. I sat on the chair beside her. My face was close to hers. I held the watch where she could see it. I held her wrist. I can still see the red of her face, the wideness of her eyes as they bulged at the enormous *size* of the pains that racked her.

Sisters came and went. They had to see how wide the cervix was. At first it was only two centimetres, not nearly enough room for you to come out. An hour later they announced it was four centimetres. It had to get to nine centimetres before we could even think of you being born. There had to be room for your head (which we had been told was big – well, we were told wrong, weren't we?) and your shoulders to slip through. It felt to your mother that this labour would go on for eight or twelve or twenty hours. That she should endure this intensity of pain for this time was unthinkable. It was like running a hundred-metre race which was stretching to ten miles. She wanted an epidural – a pain blocker.

But when the sister heard this, she said: 'Oh, do try to hang on. You're doing *so* well.'

I went to the sister, like a shop steward.

I said: 'My wife wants an epidural, so can you please arrange it?'

The sister agreed to fetch the anaesthetist, but there was between us – I admit it now – a silent conspiracy, for although I had pressed the point and she had agreed it was your mother's right, we both believed (I, for my part, on her advice) that if your mother could endure a little longer she could have the birth she wanted – without an epidural.

The anaesthetist came and went. The pain was at its worst. A midwife came and inspected your mother. She said: 'Ten centimetres.'

She said: 'Your baby is about to be born.'

We kissed, your mother and I. We kissed with soft, passionate lips as we did the day we lay on a bed at Lovett Bay and conceived you. That day the grass outside the window was a brilliant green beneath the vibrant petals of fallen jacaranda.

Outside the penumbra of our consciousness trolleys were wheeled. Sterile bags were cut open. The contractions did not stop, of course.

The obstetrician had not arrived. She was in a car, driving fast towards the hospital.

I heard a midwife say: 'Who can deliver in this position?' (It was still unusual, as I learned at that instant, for women to deliver their babies on all fours.)

Someone left the room. Someone entered. Your mother was pressing the gas mask so hard against her face it was making deep indentations on her skin. Her eyes bulged huge.

Someone said: 'Well, get her, otherwise I'll have to deliver it myself.'

The door opened. Bushfire came in.

Bushfire was Aboriginal. She was about fifty years old. She was compact and taciturn like a farmer. She had a face that folded in on itself and let out its feelings slowly, selectively. It was a face to trust, and trust especially at this moment when I looked up to see Bushfire coming through the door in a green gown. She came in a rush, her hands out to have gloves put on.

There was another contraction. I heard the latex snap around Bushfire's wrists. She said: 'There it is. I can see your baby's head.' It was you. The tip of you, the top of you. You were a new country, a planet, a star seen for the first time. I was not looking at Bushfire. I was looking at your mother. She was all alight with love and pain.

'Push,' said Bushfire.

Your mother pushed. It was you she was pushing, you that put that look of luminous love on her face, you that made the veins on her forehead bulge and her skin go red.

Then – it seems such a short time later – Bushfire said: 'Your baby's head is born.'

And then, so quickly in retrospect, but one can no more recall it accurately than one can recall exactly how one made love on a bed when the jacaranda petals were lying like jewels on the grass outside. Soon. Soon we heard you. Soon you slipped out of your mother. Soon you came slithering out not having hurt her, not even having grazed her. You slipped out, as slippery as a little fish, and we heard you cry. Your cry was so much lighter and thinner than I might have expected. I do not mean that it was weak or frail, but that your first cry had a timbre unlike anything I had expected. The joy we felt. Your mother and I kissed again, at that moment.

'My little baby,' she said. We were crying with happiness. 'My little baby.'

I turned to look. I saw you. Skin. Blue-white, shiny-wet. I said: 'It's a boy.'

'Look at me,' your mother said, meaning: stay with me, be with me, the pain is not over yet, do not leave me now. I turned to her. I kissed her. I was crying, just crying with happiness that you were there.

The room you were born in was quiet, not full of noise and clattering. This is how we wanted it for you. So you could come into the world gently and that you should – as you were now – be put on to your mother's stomach. They wrapped you up. I said: 'Couldn't he feel his mother's skin?' They unwrapped you so you could have your skin against hers.

And there you were. It was you. You had a face, the face we had never known. You were so calm. You did not cry or fret. You had big eyes like your mother's. And yet when I looked at you first I saw not your mother and me, but your two grandfathers, your mother's father, my father; and, as my father, whom I loved a great deal, had died the year before, I was moved to see that here, in you, he was alive.

Look at the photographs in the album that we took at this time. Look at your mother and how alive she is, how clear her eyes are, how all the red pain has just slipped off her face and left the unmistakable visage of a young woman in love.

We bathed you (I don't know whether this was before or after) in warm water and you accepted this gravely, swimming instinctively.

I held you (I think this must be before), and you were warm and slippery. You had not been bathed when I held you. The obstetrician gave you to me so she could examine your mother. She said: 'Here.'

I held you against me. I knew then that your mother would not die. I thought: It's fine, it's all right. I held you against my breast. You smelled of love-making.

# Pearl

## *Julia Darling*

Pearl has two faces. When she is standing on the crossing holding her lollipop stick she has a buttery smile and eyes that slant upwards. After the cars have gone she turns and her dark face with the pursed mouth and the two lines on her forehead crosses her features, like a stage curtain.

Lollipop ladies never have uniforms that fit. They always look lonely. I think of Pearl like that; as a round shape in a square world. I dream about her sometimes. Embarrassing dreams about swimming and world wars. She is in them, changing faces like the weather.

Perhaps it is the knitting.

When Pearl isn't being a lollipop lady she sits on a wall by the crossing and knits. Once I read in a newspaper about a woman who was banned from a public house for knitting in the corner. The male customers said it disturbed them. She took the manager to court and won, so I suppose the men went somewhere else. It's very hard to get to know someone who always knits, and you never know what they're thinking when they're clicking away.

I walk over the crossing every day. The walk is so boring that I can't even remember doing it some days. There is a chemist's shop, and a row of pruned trees, then the crossing, then the footpath through a dismal trodden-down park to the school gate. I see the same people each morning and afternoon, mothers mostly; barging along with prams, muttering, hunching their shoulders in the

57

wind. I don't know what they do the rest of the time. These people are stuck in my memory trudging along the pavement. We say things to each other like: 'Are we late?' or, 'Christ, it's cold!'

I am eight months' pregnant. I am dreaming most of the time. Things are very slow; very methodical. My daughter doesn't like the idea of the baby. She doesn't understand how it happened. She says it will smell. She wants me to have it adopted. I am sure that she will come round when the baby is born. We are very close.

One muddy morning we get to the crossing and Pearl says: 'Not long now!' and I sigh appropriately.

Then she rummages about in her plastic coat and pulls out something wrapped in tissue paper. Something soft.

'Open it,' says Pearl with her good face.

'Yes, open it,' says my daughter.

It is a pair of booties with little pink ribbons threaded through them. They smell of cigarettes. My daughter is enchanted. I thank Pearl twice and wander on. I can feel her watching me. I'm not sure if I behaved properly.

I don't know why, but it becomes more of an ordeal crossing the road after that. I feel I have to say something grateful. I search for pleasantries. Another mother tells me that Pearl always knits things for other people's babies.

'Isn't she kind?' says the other mother.

'Oh yes,' I agree. She is.

A week later Pearl gives me another package. This time it's a matinée jacket with mother-of-pearl buttons. It's tiny; it would fit one of my daughter's dolls. I am, of course, doubly grateful, even though I'm not all that keen on traditional baby clothes in white, pink or blue. I like to dress my babies in yellow or red.

At home I lay out the new baby's things on the floor in neat piles. I have bought some expensive soap, and a huge bra like a harness with fat straps. I have a pair of men's pyjamas to wear after the birth. I have sewn up the front. I put Pearl's presents on one side. I don't really want them.

I wonder if Pearl is curious about the father. I got the sperm through a self-help group. I administered it with a cake-icing syringe. I was incredulous when it worked. It felt like an immaculate conception. I have tried to explain it to my daughter but she looks suspicious. She's taken to talking about storks.

A week before I am due to go into labour Pearl gives me a third parcel. I open it in the rain. It is a hat with a bobble hanging from the top and two ear flaps. It must have been very difficult to knit. I thank her again, but perhaps she senses a weariness in my voice, because her dark face crosses her features like a cloud passing, and I shudder. Late pregnancy is a really peculiar state. I am so over-sensitive that anything can make me feel like crying. The hat has that effect on me. I throw it into the nearest rubbish bin and walk on guiltily.

That night my contractions start. They are like cart-horses galloping through my body. I am having a home birth. My friends loom over me with sponges and ice. The midwife has to fight her way through cheering lesbians to deliver my baby.

He is born at dawn. He cries like a blackbird. My daughter looks at her brother, clutching a baby doll. The doll is wearing Pearl's knitted clothes, just like a real baby.

Afterwards I fall asleep; hearing distant jubilation and champagne bubbling in the kitchen.

A fortnight later I am walking to school again, pushing the baby in a large and ornate pram I bought at an Oxfam shop. I am very proud of it. It has silver fittings and a navy-blue canopy with tassels. The baby looks angelic, with smooth skin and fingers that curl into tiny crescents. He is wearing a velveteen Babygro. Some of the mothers slip silver coins under the baby's rug. It is a custom round here. I nod beatifically and push on, feeling light and proud of myself. When I see Pearl she has a dark brooding expression, and I suddenly recall the hat. I smile at her hopefully. She looms over the precipice of the pram edge.

Before I even speak Pearl has picked up the baby. There is a crowd of women flapping like crows around me, watching. Pearl squeezes the baby into her coarse plastic coat and glowers. I am suddenly frightened. I step towards her. A vast lorry thunders past, splashing my legs with water.

'Give him back, Pearl,' I say loudly.

All the other mothers are cawing and crowing. I reach out to take the baby, and Pearl shakes her head and steps back. I am nearly hysterical.

Then a big mother in a mackintosh shouts militaristically: 'PUT THAT BABY DOWN!' and Pearl's face changes and she grins apologetically and puts the baby back in the pram.

'Isn't he a darling!' she says in a quite normal voice.

But the crowd of women are shaking their heads maliciously, and my daughter is crying.

When I get home I phone up the council and register a complaint. They are very soothing.

My friends come round and discuss Pearl at length. I get into bed and leave them to it. I feel obscurely guilty. I don't mention the hat.


Pearl disappears.

There is a new red-haired lollipop lady who doesn't knit and who wears wellington boots. She looks homely and rural.

As the months go by I look for Pearl. Sometimes I think I see her sad large shape passing my window, or at the far end of supermarkets. I don't forget her. She is still in my dreams.

The baby sits up now, and pummels his fists on the floor. My daughter plays with him. Her doll still wears the white bootees and the matinée jacket, although they are dirty and the wool is unravelling in some places.

One day she comes home from school with a face that is soggy with unwiped tears. When I try to comfort her she pushes me away.

'What is it?' I say, trying to be kind.

'Other kids,' she says, holding her doll as if she wants to strangle it.

'What about them?'

'They said you were a pervert.'

Of course it was bound to happen. I search them out with my eyes on the way to school and curse them.

My daughter makes me wear a dress and lipstick. I feel as if I am acting.

Increasingly, after that, I feel isolated, as if there is a subtle silence in the air. I keep my head up and walk quickly.

Months pass.

It is June when Pearl appears, and the walk to school is green and leisurely. The children are all dressed in T-shirts and shorts and climbing on the walls. I push my baby along in a buggy. He is hot and blotchy. I am beginning to consider the world beyond these small streets.

At first I don't recognise her. She is standing in the park next to a municipal rose bush licking a strawberry ice cream. She is wearing a summer hat and looking undeniably handsome. Her other hand rests on the bar of a spanking new pram.

At first I turn the other way, thinking that I will make a detour around the sandpit to avoid colliding with her on the narrow path, then my daughter says loudly: 'There's Pearl,' and she looks up and sees us.

She waves.

I am very embarrassed then, even afraid of her, but I walk towards her, driven by curiosity.

As we get nearer she gives a proud, royal nod, and I smile bravely, suddenly remembering that I should slip a silver coin into the pram for a new baby.

'Hello, Pearl,' I say conversationally, gripping a fifty-pence piece in my hand.

My son giggles and points at Pearl's hat.

'He's grown,' she says, her face a crease of smiles.

I lean over the pram indulgently, and pull back the cotton sheet.

The first thing I see is a white knitted hat with ear flaps, neatly tied around a small head. I lean in further.

'What's its name?' asks my daughter.

Pearl pauses, then says, 'It's a she.'

I see the baby's face then. It is small and perfect, beautifully crafted in skin-coloured wool.

Pearl has knitted herself a baby.

My mouth hangs open. I struggle for words, but she has turned on her heels and is walking across the park, away from me, disappearing into a leafy avenue of trees, like a spell.

# Deliverance
## *Judith Bryan*

*First Stage*

Sciatica came first, a warning to take nothing for granted. It seized me one evening on my way home from work. A colleague sidled me across the pavement inch by inch, like a washing machine being moved across the kitchen floor, and levered me into a taxi. I was only three months 'gone', just beginning to show but already waddling. Beneath my clothes, my bump lay hard and intense, smooth as a lychee seed.

Then, a few weeks later, the stretchmarks started. As a faithful devotee of body lotion, I'd never had any before. Besides, my mother, who'd borne three children in five years, had no more lines on her belly than on her soft brown face. 'We have elastic skin in our family,' she'd always say, giving her stomach a complacent little pat before wriggling into her panty girdle. 'Not bad for a sixty year old.' At the age of thirty, I was pregnant with my first child. And I was not like my mother.

The stretchmarks came at a rate of about three a week. I felt the slow rip of each one as it was born. Starting as a hot, itchy spot in my epidermis, they crept relentlessly across my stomach like ladders in a pair of tights. They went down to my pubic hair and up to my navel. Sometimes they branched out or broke off or two ran side by side, competing with each other. The bigger I got, the more adventurous they became. Snail trails swirled around my belly. The stretched skin was beautiful, translucent bronze markings on a brown dome. It shimmered and sang. It bloody hurt.

I switched from body lotion to cocoa butter, applying copious amounts. A warm spring was followed by a hot summer and my extra high, pregnant-body heat conspired with the weather to melt the cocoa butter. My skin was slick with it; I gave off delicious, mouthwatering fumes and I felt gorgeous, glowing, like a vast, ripe fruit. At the health centre, the nurse grimaced every time she touched me. Her hand came away shiny, bits of my skin peppering her palm. Finally she asked, 'Did you wash this morning?' and I hated her, violently.

The cocoa butter didn't work, of course. Again I was reminded: take nothing for granted, neither inherited skin tone nor what my sisters fondly called my 'childbearing hips'. This, all this, was pregnancy – a process I could not control. My body could do any of the things I'd read about in endless pregnancy manuals. Or it could do none of them; it could invent new things to do.

But warnings were for wimps; I ignored them and went my merry way, acquiescent partner in tow. Geraint nodded and smiled and did the cooking. I was nauseous and couldn't bear to cook, not just for twelve weeks but for the entire pregnancy. My job was Planning. Early on, I had decided against a hospital birth. I wanted an alternative delivery at home, with a water pool and the minimum of intervention. Soon after the sciatica incident I started ante-natal yoga classes at the Active Birth Centre. And I read, obsessively – everything from Sheila Kitzinger to Dr Jolly.

Of the four home-birth midwives, Margaret was my favourite. From the moment she walked into our living room, I felt safe with her. Dressed in bright T-shirts, leggings and big dangly earrings she managed to be both wonderfully informal and totally professional. One afternoon we shared a girly moan about the perils of weight gain in later life. (Despite my nausea, I'd managed to put on three stone, which helped neither the sciatica nor the stretchmarks.)

'I just keep getting bigger and bigger,' she said, 'but I'm in the gym four nights a week. Feel my thigh.'

I gave it a gentle poke, suddenly aware that this woman was more than my midwife, she was my friend. Her leg was solid as a rock, a metaphor for Margaret herself. After all the careful planning, the one thing we wouldn't need was the birth-plan itself. Margaret was simpatico. In her hands, all would be well. By the time my maternity leave started, four weeks before my due date, I felt in control again. All that remained was to book the pool and work out how to fill it.

Halfway through my maternity leave, Margaret took a week's holiday. I wasn't to worry, she said, she'd be at home and I was to ask the team to call her if I started early. At the next visit Alice came. We went through the drill: sonic aid, blood pressure and urine test. My blood pressure was a little high, not worryingly so but we'd have to watch it. I lay languidly occupying the window seat as Alice gazed down at me.

'Have you been exerting yourself?' she asked dubiously. Actually, I'd been weeding the front garden. Geraint and I had never minded having a thistle jungle outside our front-room window but suddenly, that morning, it had seemed terribly important to clear it.

'You're going to have to take it a bit easy.'

But I had the airing cupboard to tidy, new baby clothes to wash and our bedroom to finish decorating . . .

Because of the raised blood pressure, Alice came again the following day. Sonic aid, blood pressure, urine test: I heaved myself up the stairs to the toilet, returning with the limp litmus strip for her to check against her chart. Alice winced. She held the chart up for me to see.

'I'm sorry,' she said, 'there are traces of protein in your urine. You're going to have to go into hospital. Today. Now. You've developed pre-eclampsia.'

## Second Stage

It was nice at first. I was in for a rest. The doctor said I had none of the associated symptoms of pre-eclampsia – headache, altered vision, abdominal pain. In fact, I felt so well I simply couldn't accept that there was anything wrong with me or the baby. Still, there was something quite comforting about being in hospital. Geraint came with fruit, magazines, kisses. I was free to lie about doing nothing. Like the ward's orange curtains that filtered the heat, the nurses were jolly. I spent a night in a comfy hospital bed feeling calm and at peace.

In the morning, around the time that Geraint would have already left the house for work, another doctor came. My blood pressure was still rising, she said, despite the night's rest. With this condition it would keep on rising. She reminded me that pre-eclampsia could be fatal, for both mother and child. The only cure was to have the baby. It was in my best interests to have an induced labour. It would be reckless, she said, to refuse.

The bed in the labour ward was the exact height, width and firmness of an ironing board. They balanced me on the top with a continuous fetal monitor strapped across my stomach, a blood-pressure monitor on my arm and injunctions not to move. The machines were sensitive: undue movement could confuse the readings. Hospital midwives came, serious-faced, abrupt women who seemed to prefer not to meet my eyes. They prodded my ankles,

66

hands and face for oedema, examined me internally, took blood tests. A third doctor came. He managed to insert an intravenous valve into the back of my hand whilst completely ignoring me.

'Ow,' I said. 'That hurts.'

Rather than acknowledge my comment he looked over his shoulder, exchanging medical jargon with the nurse at the other end of the room. The needle in the IV valve felt like a Stanley knife scraping across my veins. When he had finished, he glanced at me for the first time, a small smile lifting his lips.

I held on to the tears until the nurse and doctor left. My sobs sounded strange in the sparse, square room, echoing off the white walls, counterpoint to the beep of the fetal monitor. I felt stranded, stunned. I wished Margaret was there to guide me, or Geraint to hold my hand, but there was only me and the baby. Would it resent being hurried into the world, forced out with drugs and surrounded by strangers? Or was it in trouble, desperate to leave but being slowly killed by the chemical reaction between my body and its own? My hand throbbed. Gingerly, I rubbed the area around the IV valve. This was not the labour I had planned. I won't let them treat me this way, I thought angrily. I'll discharge myself, go home and phone Margaret, give birth in the bath . . .

The fetal monitor beeped on. It produced slow scrolls of paper etched with indecipherable markings. These inky scribbles, with their odd stalagmites and stalactites, were my baby's heartbeats. My baby's breath and movements, its life. Inducing labour meant that I could hold that life in my arms, not in two weeks' time but today. I stopped crying and watched the erratic black lines dance up and down the paper.

'Miss Bryan?' Another nurse entered the room. She held up a surgical dish piled with packages. 'I've come to insert the prostin gel into your cervix. Are you ready?' Her voice was kind and she was smiling. Smiling back, I wiped the tears from my face.

'Yes, I'm ready.'

The prostin, like the cocoa butter, didn't work. By evening I was back on the ward with the orange curtains. Geraint came in with my bean bag, just in case. More importantly, he brought Kentucky Fried Chicken. Hidden by the bed screen, we crunched bones and chuckled. The baby didn't want to come! It was obviously fine, impervious to the hospital's potions, biding its time. Geraint wiped the grease off his mouth with a paper napkin.

'Even so,' he said, 'why don't we call Margaret in?'

But now that the drama was over, I demurred. I didn't want to make a fuss. I said, 'She's entitled to a bit of peace on her holiday.'

At this point Geraint was supposed to insist, like men do in romantic novels: 'Nonsense, darling. It's Margaret you need and it's Margaret you shall have.' Instead he scrumpled the napkin between his hands and pulled something out of his rucksack. 'In that case, we'd better fill this in. It's the birth-plan. I think we're going to need it.'

He was right, of course. Twenty-four hours and two plugs of prostin later, I was strapped to the ironing board again. There were some weak contractions and a lot of backache but I wasn't in labour. Meanwhile, my friend the fetal monitor was becoming treacherous: the scribbly stalagmites kept going flat.

'It might be the machine,' a nurse said.

I was surprised to hear her admit it. We'd been told about the notorious unreliability of fetal monitors in Active Birth classes – the machines go skew-whiff, the hospital staff panic, before you know where you are you're flat on your back with an epidural, unable to move from the chest down.

'On the other hand,' she added, balancing skeins of paper between her palms, 'the baby might be in distress.'

By midnight, the baby wasn't the only one. Apart from being woken every forty minutes for a vaginal exam or blood-pressure reading, or just to find out if I was 'comfortable', I'd tried to go for a wee at half past eleven and found I couldn't. I felt decidedly full but nothing came out. Catheter, the doctor said. Over my dead body, I said, remembering the pain of the IV valve. They'd have to tie me down before I let them put tubes into me. I started to cry. The doctor exchanged irritated looks with the nurse.

'We'll leave you for an hour,' she said darkly, 'but after that we're going to have to do something.'

At half past twelve a relief nurse came. 'Well then, let's get you a jug of water,' she said cheerfully, 'and see what happens.'

An hour later I was crouched over a bed pan, pissing like a horse.

At three a.m. the alarm went on the blood-pressure monitor. The nurses rushed in, fiddling with knobs and wires. This is it, I thought, emergency Caesarean time. They're going to wheel me off to the operating theatre. But it was the machine that got wheeled off. It *was* faulty. Soon after, as if on cue, contractions finally started. Every three to four minutes, for about half a minute. The ironing board was like a bed of nails beneath me. Lying still was a physical impossibility. Heedless of the nurses' protests, I swung my legs over the side and headed for the bean bag.

I wanted Geraint with me but they said it was too soon, I wasn't in real labour yet. It felt real enough to me. At six o'clock they relented. By quarter past he was there, massaging my back and exhorting me to breathe. It was then, for the first time, that I felt excited. This was hyper-real, like the movies or in books. Breathe, says the husband, breathe. The woman moans, the machine bleeps, and the nurses do efficient things with obscure-looking equipment.

Then the morning-shift nurse came. Her preferred equipment was her hand. She put on a latex glove and advanced towards me, offering to rupture my membranes. The doctor had suggested it but our birth-plan emphatically excluded this procedure. I told her so. She wasn't giving up that easy.

'OK, Mum,' she said, 'I'll just give you an internal exam, then. We need to measure your cervix and find out where Baby's head is.'

It was very odd being called Mum whilst being treated like a particularly stupid child. Still, I hadn't had an internal since the contractions started; I was curious to know how dilated I was. With Geraint's help, I got back on the ironing board. The nurse smiled, a grim, private smile. The gloved hand dived under my hospital gown and . . .

'Jesus!' It was all I could do not to kick her in the face. It was as if she was rooting around in there with that Stanley knife.

'Hold on,' she said. 'I just need to –'

'Stop it!' Geraint yelled. 'You're hurting her!'

He tried to pull me away but I couldn't move. It was like being in the jaws of a crocodile. I was screaming and crying and at last she backed off, holding her hand at head height like a trophy. I tumbled off the bed, weak at the knees, Geraint's arms around me, and my waters broke – a gush of clear fluid pooling over the floor.

For months I'd fantasised about my waters breaking: where it would happen, how it would feel, the drama of calling out the midwife, filling the pool, getting everything ready. Over Geraint's shoulder I saw the nurse, smirking by the door. I was 99 per cent certain she had done it on purpose, but my overriding feeling was one of relief. It was as if my body had been given a second chance. Maybe now the rest would happen naturally. At that moment the door opened. The nurse ripped off her glove, looking guilty. A familiar face peered into the room, assessing the situation in a moment.

'Hello,' said Margaret. 'All ready to go then, are we?'

The hospital staff melted away, like ghouls in a nightmare. Margaret bustled into action, scolding us for not calling her in. Alice had told her that morning, otherwise she would have come as soon as I was admitted. Straight away, she began to negotiate behind the scenes on my behalf. Of course I could have a mattress on the floor if that was what I wanted. And yes, the doctor would consider allowing me to use the hospital's fitted birth-pool if my blood pressure stabilised. Margaret suggested a shot of pethidine to help with the pain. After that I lay on the mattress in a pleasant stupor, a towel under one hip and a hot-water bottle balanced on the other. The contractions crunched into my pelvis, tensing my stomach and making my legs wobble. It was an interesting sensation but not painful, as if it was happening to someone else. I drifted into sleep, listening to Margaret and Geraint talking quietly nearby.

When I woke up, my mum was there. Without my glasses on, she was blurry round the edges. Which, perhaps, was just as well. She was completely naked except for her panty girdle and she was doing a hula-hula dance. She took hold of the girdle's waistband and rolled it down. Her belly button popped into view, then, bit by bit, the rest of her.

'See this stomach?' she crowed. 'Pristine! And just to think, I'll be sixty-one years old next birthday.'

I closed my eyes. The next time I opened them she was sitting a few feet away, her handbag perched on her knee, wearing a sun hat and her summer mac. She saw me looking at her and winked. This pethidine is good stuff, I thought.

'Hi, Mum,' I said, not believing for a minute that she was really there.

'Hi, darling,' she said. 'How're you doing?'

Geraint loomed into my field of vision. 'I told her not to come all this way but you know your mum. She said she wouldn't miss her first grandchild being born for the world.'

An hour later the contractions were coming stronger, lasting twice as long. I got up on all fours and laid my head in my mum's lap. She stroked my hair, crooning tunelessly, and it soothed me. Geraint came to massage my back. Suddenly his touch felt heavy, jarring. Hissing, I shrugged him off. He retreated to a corner and I heard Margaret say something about 'second stage'.

'Can you feel yourself opening?'

She spoke loudly as if calling to me from another country. Blearily, I gazed in her direction. 'Yes, yes, I'm opening. Like a flower. Like a rose.'

From the distant shores of Labour I saw her glance up at my mum, a crooked grin on her face. She took my blood pressure, then I felt rummaging going on under my gown again.

'Four or five centimetres,' Margaret announced. 'What do you think, Judith – still want to try the water-bath?'

*Third Stage*

The pastel-coloured room glowed with subdued light. Light reflected off the water and snaked across framed prints on the walls. The pool – twice the size of anything I could have booked for use at home – was filled and ready. The water formed a dark circle, lapping gently against the sides. Geraint and my mum each held one of my elbows and we stumbled across the floor. I chuckled to myself as they helped me up and into the pool. I felt a right old fraud, wilting theatrically like James Brown, a towel draped over my shoulders and sweat trickling down my temples. Still, they had to hold tight to stop me falling in as my legs collapsed beneath me. The warm water came to just under my breasts. On one side was a broad shelf for me to rest on. Smiling and sighing, I lay back. Warily, Geraint moved in behind me and put his arms around me. His touch felt good again. Almost at once I began to doze.

The contractions woke me. Margaret said I should stand, so at each one I swung myself up, knock-kneed in the water. When it had passed I subsided, exhausted, happily convinced that it was the last pain, and fell immediately to sleep again. This went on for two hours. The water tumbled around the dome of my stomach, dissolving me in its darkness. I could hardly feel my body; I was just a belly, clenching and unclenching. It got harder to wake up. Geraint's hands slipped on my wet skin and I went from standing to merely lurching around. I was a hippo in a hollow. I started grunting, muted booms in the echoey room, like a heartbeat under water, like the baby's heartbeat through ultrasound.

I heard Margaret calling my name. 'Look at me!' She put her hands on either side of my face and fixed me in her gaze. 'It's time to push,' she said.

The prevailing wisdom was for mothers to exit the pool at this stage in the labour, so that babies wouldn't actually be born in water. A high bed, very like the object of my earlier torture, waited on the other side of the room. But to leave the pool now would seem like a punishment. As well as feeling I hadn't the strength to move, I had a sudden conviction that the birth was going to take another un-expected turn. In the past few hours I'd become compla-cent, forgetting the lesson of the sciatica, the stretchmarks, the pre-eclampsia: take nothing for granted. Margaret must have seen the panic in my face.

'It's all right,' she said. 'We can do it right here.' She gestured to Geraint and, with his help, I stood again.

'Push.'

'Blow.'

I felt the head crowning, felt myself stretching. Every sensation was suddenly concentrated into the area around the baby's head.

'I can't do it, it burns.'

I started to tip my head back, my mouth widening for a scream, but Margaret wasn't having it.

'Look at me, Judith!' Our eyes made four again, locked tight and, like a lighthouse in the fog, her gaze and voice steered me safe. 'You can do it. Push. Now blow, blow, blow.'

The burn was exquisite, beyond pain, and then I felt a sort of pop, a release of tension. I slid back into the water, felt him slither away from me, turning as he went down. I laughed. My voice rang loud. Down he went, then up, up like a pearl diver, lifted in Margaret's hands. Water streamed from his body, running off her elbows. She put him in my arms. His little grey face gazed up at me, onyx-eyed. We bobbed together on the water, Geraint leaning over my shoulder, embracing us both.

'So that's what you look like,' I said. 'Hello, Baby.'

# The Snapper (extract)

## *Roddy Doyle*

– You're wha'? said Jimmy Rabbitte Sr.

He said it loudly.

– You heard me, said Sharon.

Jimmy Jr was upstairs in the boys' room doing his DJ practice. Darren was in the front room watching *Police Academy II* on the video. Les was out. Tracy and Linda, the twins, were in the front room annoying Darren. Veronica, Mrs Rabbitte, was sitting opposite Jimmy Sr at the kitchen table.

Sharon was pregnant and she'd just told her father that she thought she was. She'd told her mother earlier, before the dinner.

– Oh – my Jaysis, said Jimmy Sr.

He looked at Veronica. She looked tired. He looked at Sharon again.

– That's shockin', he said.

Sharon said nothing.

– Are yeh sure? said Jimmy Sr.

– Yeah. Sort of.

– Wha'?

– Yeah.

Jimmy Sr wasn't angry. He probably wouldn't be either, but it all seemed very unfair.

– You're only nineteen, he said.

– I'm twenty.

– You're only twenty.

– I know what age I am, Daddy.

– Now, there's no need to be gettin' snotty, said Jimmy Sr.

– Sorry, said Sharon.

She nearly meant it.

– I'm the one tha' should be gettin' snotty, said Jimmy Sr.

Sharon made herself smile. She was happy with the way things were going so far.

– It's shockin', said Jimmy Sr again, – so it is. Wha' do you think o' this?

He was talking to Veronica.

– I don't know, said Veronica.

– Is tha' the best yeh can do, Veronica?

– Well, what do YOU think?

Jimmy Sr creased his face and held it that way for a second.

– I don't know, he said. – I should give ou', I suppose. An' throw a wobbler or somethin'. But – what's the point?

Veronica nodded. She looked very tired now.

Jimmy Sr continued.

– If she was –

He turned to Sharon.

– You should've come to us earlier – before, yeh know – an' said you were goin' to get pregnant.

The three of them tried to laugh.

– Then we could've done somethin' abou' it. – My God, though.

No one said anything. Then Jimmy Sr spoke to Sharon again.

– You're absolutely sure now? Positive?

– Yeah, I am. I done –

– Did, said Veronica.

– I did the test.

– The test? said Jimmy Sr. – Oh. – Did yeh go in by yourself?

76

– Yeah, said Sharon.

– Did yeh? Fair play to yeh, said Jimmy Sr. – I'd never've thought o' tha'.

Sharon and Veronica looked at each other, and grinned quickly.

Jimmy Sr got down to business.

– Who was it?

– Wha'? – Oh. I don't know.

– Ah now, Jaysis –!

– No, I do know.

– Well, then?

– I'm not tellin'.

Jimmy Sr could feel himself getting a bit angry now. That was better.

– Now, look –

They heard Jimmy Jr from up in the boys' room.

– THIS IS JIMMY RABBITTE – ALL – OVER – IRELAND.

– Will yeh listen to tha' fuckin' eejit, said his father.

– Leave him alone, said Veronica.

Jimmy Sr stared at the ceiling.

– I don't know.

Then he turned to Sharon again.

– Why won't yeh tell us?

Sharon said nothing. Jimmy Sr saw her eyes filling with water.

– Don't start tha', he told her. – Just tell us.

– I can't, Sharon told the table.

– Why not?

– I just can't, righ'.

Jimmy Sr looked across at Veronica and shook his head. He'd never been able to cope with answers like that. If Sharon had been one of the boys he'd have walloped her.

Veronica looked worried now. She wasn't sure she really wanted to know the answer.

– Is he married? Jimmy Sr asked.

– Oh my God, said Veronica.

– No, he's not! said Sharon.

– Well, that's somethin', I suppose, said Jimmy Sr. –
Then why –

Veronica started crying.

– Ah Veronica, stop tha'.

Linda ran in.

– Daddy, Darren's after hittin' me.

She was getting ready to cry.

– Jesus! Another one, said Jimmy Sr.

Then he spoke to Linda.

– I'll go in in a minute an' I'll hit Darren an' you can
watch me hittin' him.

– Can I?

– Yeah, yeh can. Now get ou' or I'll practise on you first.

Linda squealed and ran away from him. She stopped at
the safe side of the kitchen door.

– Can Tracy watch as well? she asked.

– She can o' course. Now, your mammy an' Sharon an'
me are havin' a chat, so leave us alone.

Jimmy Sr looked at the two women. The crying had
stopped.

– THIS IS JIMMY RABBITTE – ALL – OVER – IRELAND.

– Oh good Jesus, what a house! – Is he queer or wha' is
he? Jimmy Sr asked Sharon.

– No, he's not. He's alrigh'; leave him alone.

– I don't know, said Jimmy Sr. – Tha' gear he wears. He
had his trous –

– That's only the fashion.

– I suppose so. But, Jaysis.

He looked at Veronica. She just looked tired again.

– This is an awful shock, Sharon, he said. – Isn't it,
Veronica?

– Definitely.

– Make us a cup o' tea there, love, will yeh.

78

– Make it yourself, said Veronica.

– I'll make it, said Sharon.

– Good girl, said Jimmy Sr. – Mind yourself against the table there. Good girl. – You're sure now he's not married?

– Yeah, he's not, said Sharon, at the sink.

– Then why won't yeh tell us then?

– Look, said Sharon.

She turned to face him.

– I can't, an' I'm not goin' to.

She turned back to plug in the kettle.

– Will he marry you? Jimmy Sr asked her.

– No. I don't think so.

– The louser. That's cheatin', tha' is.

– It's not a game! said Veronica.

– I know, I know tha', Veronica. But it's his fault as much as Sharon's. Whoever he is. – It was his flute tha' –

– Daddy!

– Well, it was.

– It's no wonder they all talk the way they do, Veronica gave out to Jimmy Sr.

– Ah, lay off, Veronica, will yeh.

They heard a scream from the front room.

– Hang on till I sort this young fella ou', said Jimmy Sr. He marched out of the kitchen.

– He's taking it well, said Veronica.

– Yeah, said Sharon. – So are you.

– Ah sure –

– I was afraid you'd throw me ou'.

– I never thought of that, mind you. – It's not right though, said Veronica.

She looked straight at Sharon.

– I suppose it's not, said Sharon.

Jimmy Sr came back, rubbing his hands and calling Darren a sneaky little bastard. He sat down and saw the tea waiting for him.

– Aah, lovely.

He sipped.

– Fuck! – Sorry, Veronica; excuse me. It's very hot.

– He's started saying Excuse me. After twenty-two years.

– Good luck, Jimmy Jr roared from the front door, and then he slammed it.

– He shuts the door like a normal man annyway. That's somethin', I suppose.

– He's alrigh', said Sharon.

Jimmy Sr now said something he'd heard a good few times on the telly.

– D'yeh want to keep it?

– Wha' d'yeh mean?

– D'yeh – d'you want to keep it, like?

– He wants to know if you want to have an abortion, said Veronica. – The eejit.

– I do not! said Jimmy Sr.

This was true. He was sorry now he'd said it.

– There's no way I'd have an abortion, said Sharon.

– Good. You're right.

– Abortion's murder.

– It is o' course.

Then he thought of something and he had to squirt his tea back into the cup. He could hear his heart. And feel it.

He looked at Sharon.

– He isn't a black, is he?

– No!

He believed her. The three of them started laughing.

– One o' them students, yeh know, Jimmy Sr explained. – With a clatter o' wives back in Africa.

– Stop that.

Jimmy Sr's tea was finished.

– That was grand, Sharon, thanks, he said. – An' you're def'ny not goin' to tell us who it is?

– No. – Sorry.

– Never mind the Sorry. – I think you should tell us. I'm not goin' to kill him or annythin'.

Sharon said nothing.

Jimmy Sr pushed his chair back from the table.

– There's no point in anny more talkin' then, I suppose. Your mind's obviously made up, Sharon.

He stood up.

– A man needs a pint after all tha', he said.

– Is that all? said Veronica, shocked.

– Wha' d'yeh mean, Veronica?

– It's a terrible – Veronica started.

But she couldn't really go on. She thought that Sharon's news deserved a lot more attention, and some sort of punishment. As far as Veronica was concerned this was the worst thing that had ever happened to the family. But she couldn't really explain why, not really. And she knew that, anyway, nothing could be done about it. Maybe it wouldn't be so bad once she got used to it.

Then she thought of something.

– The neighbours, she said.

– Wha' abou' them? said Jimmy Sr.

Veronica thought for a bit.

– What'll they say? she then said.

– You don't care wha' tha' lot says, do yeh? said Jimmy Sr.

– Yes. I do.

– Ah now, Veronica.

He sat down.

Sharon spoke.

– They'll have a laugh when they find ou' an' they'll try an' guess who I'm havin' it for. An' that's all. – An' anyway, I don't care.

– An' that's the important thing, Jimmy Sr told Veronica.

Veronica didn't look convinced.

– Sure look, said Jimmy Sr. – The O'Neill young ones have had kids, the both o' them. An' – an' the Bells would be the same 'cept they don't have anny daughters, but yeh know wha' I mean.

– Dawn O'Neill had her baby for Paddy Bell, Sharon reminded him.

– She did o' course, said Jimmy Sr.

He stood up.

– So there now, Veronica, he said. – Fuck the neighbours.

Veronica tried to look as if she'd been won over. She wanted to go up to bed. She nodded.

Jimmy Sr had a nice idea.

– Are yeh comin' for a drink, Sharon?

– No thanks, Daddy. I'll stay in tonigh'.

– Ah, go on.

– All righ', Sharon smiled.

– Good girl. Yeh may as well – Veronica?

– 'M? – Ah no, no thanks.

– Go on.

– No. I'm goin' up to bed.

– I'd go up with yeh only I've a throat on me.

Veronica smiled.

– You're sure now? said Jimmy Sr.

– Yep, said Veronica.

Sharon went for her jacket.

– Will I bring yeh home a few chips? Jimmy Sr asked Veronica.

– I'll be asleep.

– Fair enough.

– Jimmy Sr stopped at the front door and roared back to Veronica.

– Cheerio now, Granny.

Then he laughed, and slammed the door harder than Jimmy Jr had.

\*      \*      \*

Jimmy Sr came back with the drinks and sat in beside Sharon. He hated the tables up here, in the lounge. You couldn't get your legs in under them. Sharon couldn't either. She sat side-saddle.

– Thanks a lot, Daddy, said Sharon when she'd poured the Coke in with the vodka.

– Ah, no problem, said Jimmy Sr.

He'd never had a drink with Sharon before. He watched his pint settling, something he never did when he was downstairs in the bar. He only came up here on Sundays, and now.

He turned to Sharon and spoke softly.

– When's it due an' annyway?

– November.

Jimmy Sr did a few quick sums in his head.

– You're three months gone.

– No. Nearly.

– Yeh should've told us earlier.

– I know. – I was scared to.

– Ah, Sharon. – I still think you should tell us who the da is.

– You can think away then.

Jimmy Sr couldn't help grinning. She'd always been like that.

– I thought your mammy took it very well, he said.

– Yeah, Sharon agreed. – She was great.

– Cos she's a bit ol' fashioned like tha'. Set in her ways.

– Yeah. No, she was great. So were you.

– Ah, now.

They said nothing after that for a bit. Jimmy Sr could think of nothing else to say. He looked around him: kids and yuppies. He sat there, feeling far from home. The lads would all be downstairs by now. Jimmy Sr had a good one he'd heard in work for them, about a harelip in a sperm-bank. He loved Sharon but, if the last five minutes were anything to go by, she was shocking drinking company.

He noticed Jimmy Jr up at the stools with his pals.

— There's Jimmy, he said.

— Yeah, said Sharon.

— That's an awful-lookin' shower he hangs around with.

— They're all righ'.

— The haircuts on them, look.

— That's only the fashion these days. Leave them alone.

— I s'pose so, said Jimmy Sr.

And they stopped again.

There was only an hour to closing time but Jimmy Sr wasn't sure he'd be able to stick it.

— Wha' does Jimmy be doin' up there when he's shoutin', yeh know, abou' bein' all over Ireland? he asked Sharon.

— He wants to be a DJ.

— A wha'?

— A DJ. A disc jockey.

— Wha', like Larry Gogan?

— Yeah. Sort of.

— Jaysis, said Jimmy Sr.

He'd had enough.

He'd spotted a gang of Sharon's friends over past Jimmy Jr and his pals.

— There's those friends o' yours, Sharon, he said.

Sharon knew what he was at.

— Oh yeah, she said.

— D'yeh want to go over to them?

— I don't mind.

— They'd be better company than your oul' fella annyway, wha'.

— Ah no.

— Go on. Yeh may as well go over. I don't mind.

— I can't leave you on your own.

– Ah sure, said Jimmy Sr. – I can go down an' see if there's annyone downstairs.

Sharon grinned. So did Jimmy Sr. He still felt guilty though, so he got a fiver out and handed it to Sharon.

– Ah, there's no need, Daddy.

– There is o' course, said Jimmy Sr.

He moved in closer to her.

– It's not every day yeh find ou' you're goin' to be a granda.

He'd just thought of that now and he had to stop himself from letting his eyes water. He often did things like that, gave away pounds and fivers or said nice things; little things that made him like himself.

He patted Sharon's shoulder. He was standing up, but he stopped.

– Hang on a sec, he said. – I'll wait till your man passes.

Sharon looked.

– Who?

– Burgess there, the bollix. Excuse me, Sharon. I can't stand him.

– I've seen yeh talkin' to him loads o' times.

– He traps me. An' Darren's his goalie this year. He'd drop him if I got snotty with him.

– Oh. Yeah.

– It's all righ' now, said Jimmy Sr, and he stood up again. – The coast's clear. See yeh later.

Jimmy Sr trotted out, and down to the lads in the bar. Sharon took her vodka and her jacket and her bag and went across to Jackie O'Keefe, Mary Curran and Yvonne Burgess, her friends; the gang.

– Hiyis, she said when she got there.

– Oh, howyeh, Sharon.

– Hiyeh, Sharon.

– Howyeh, Sharon.

– Hiyis, said Sharon.

– Put your bag over here, Sharon, look, said Yvonne.

– Thanks, said Sharon. – Hiyeh, Jackie. Haven't seen yeh in ages.

– She's been busy, said Mary.

Yvonne sniggered.

– How's Greg? Sharon asked Jackie.

Yvonne sniggered again.

– Fuck off, you, said Jackie. – He's grand, Sharon.

– They're goin' on their holliers together, Mary told Sharon.

– Dirty bitch, said Yvonne.

They laughed.

– Fuck off, will yeh, said Jackie. – We're not goin' for definite.

She explained.

– He mightn't be able to take the time off.

– Yeh see, Sharon, said Yvonne. – You've got to understand, Greg's a very important person.

– Fuck off, Burgess, said Jackie, but she was grinning.

– Where're yeh goin'? Sharon asked Jackie.

– Rimini. In Italy.

– Lovely.

– Yeah.

– Yeh can go for a swim with the Pope, said Yvonne.

They laughed.

– Cos there'll be fuck all else to do there, Yvonne finished.

– She's just jealous, said Mary.

– Of wha'? said Yvonne.

Mary changed the subject.

– Anny news, Sharon? she asked.

– No, said Sharon. – Not really.

# The Twilight Zone

## *Jill Dawson*

I wake to the sound of a baby crying and realise that it's coming from the plastic box alongside my bed. Propping myself up on one elbow I lean over to take a peek, half expecting to see straw, not hospital blankets. Something is moving in there, kicking at the yellow waffle coverlet, tossing a tiny teddy into the air. The howling is a brand-new sound to me – bird-like, surreal. A bald cry, Sylvia Plath called it, clear vowels, rising like balloons to the ceiling. (How clever poetry is, to wait in the wings like that for fifteen years, just until you need it.)

'Pick him up then, Mum – or are you going to let him scream the place down?'

*Mum*. The young nurse who looms at me, with her less than friendly stage whisper, has no idea that the word has not attached itself to me. That I can't think of myself as Mum yet, after only . . . (a glance at the clock above her desk tells me it's midnight) eight hours and three minutes.

Her heels tap away down the sleeping ward. It hurts to lean over. I can't say *where* it hurts as the lower part of my body no longer belongs to me: my legs are joined together in a mermaid's tail, an after-effect of the epidural. With an effort, I manage to pluck the screaming creature from his crib, feeling his ribs all the way through the blanket, teeny bird bones wrapped in soft white towelling. I think of twiglets, feet on leaves, small snapping things. I'm terri-fied.

At the approach of my nipple, the strange baby arches his back, pulls his chin towards his neck like a tortoise drawing itself into its shell, and screams harder.

In a feeble voice, I try calling for the nurse. 'Can I have a drink of water, please?' She can't hear me over the baby's screams, sits at her desk under a yellow lamp, flicking through *Take a Break*. I'm startled by my thirst. I've never felt a thirst like this before. How curious: a raging thirst steals into me, each time the baby's mouth approaches my nipple.

*I don't know who this little person is; he wasn't here yesterday.* The baby stiffens each time I offer him my breast. His face is red and angry, hungry, demented. The woman in the bed beside mine has woken up and scowls at me, her own baby sleeping beautifully in the plastic cot beside her.

The creature in my arms thrashes and screams as if I was trying to murder him, not feed him. The nurse finally looks over at me, comes wearily to stand beside the bed. With no warning she grabs at my breast and, holding the baby's head, shoves the two together. I picture a kiss. Teenagers kissing. If you smack two mouths together, it must work. But it doesn't, of course. He pulls his head back uttering furious shrieks.

'I've tried that! He doesn't want it,' I say.

'Of course he wants it. He's hungry, poor little mite.'

Two other babies further down the ward begin crying too. Like animals, wolves howling in sympathy. The young nurse picks up my baby (is he 'my baby'? that phrase is new, too) and puts his head on her shoulder. Pats his back. Walks back towards her desk, rocking him. He draws his legs up to his knees but the howls lessen in volume, become less outraged. He begins to sound a little half-hearted. Casual even. He sounds to me like someone who could stop crying, if he really wanted to.

Finally, thankfully, he falls silent. The nurse gets up and walks back to me. Without saying a word, she puts the baby in my arms. I look at his closed mouth and he smiles in his sleep, eyeballs flickering alarmingly.

'I hate the way babies sound. Like the cats that used to yowl outside our house when I was a kid. Makes me want to throw a bucket of water at him!'

She looks at me oddly. Draws her brows together, so that the bindi in her forehead disappears between her frown. I stop talking. Instead, I allow her to take him out of my arms and place him in the crib, cover him with the blankets. How many babies has she looked after in this way? How efficient she is, how good at it all. As she walks away she steps on the abandoned teddy. It gives a forlorn little squeak.

*And will you take this baby away, please. He doesn't like me and I can tell he wants to go back.*

She doesn't turn around.

In the early hours of the morning I wake again, floating to the surface of a dream in the too-hot, airless hospital bed. For some reason, instead of crying in his plastic crib my son is right beside me in the bed, his warm limbs seeping into my skin, one tagged leg stretching in front of him. *Baby boy of Paula Jones.* He is wide awake and staring at me with a look more curious than any I've ever seen. His eyes are two tiny silver fish shimmering in a net and when I lean over to look at him he smiles at me and says: 'Hello.' I glance around the ward; tears spring into my eyes. The other women are sleeping. No one is looking at us so I put my face close to his, smelling his new-bread smell in the midst of the sterile bed and I whisper in astonishment, 'Hello, Finn,' right back.

The next morning Simon arrives, dutifully clutching a carrier bag from Boots, with things I should have put in my hospital bag – all the things the baby magazines recommended and I was convinced I could do without. He sits on the bottom of my bed, unshaven, looking absolutely, incandescently gorgeous with dark moons under his eyes and his perfect Roman nose and his Camper shoes. Brand-new shoes that he must have bought yesterday and must have cost him a bomb.

'Did you go out celebrating?'

He kisses my cheek. 'It was odd to go out without you, after so much excitement yesterday. Without you both,' he tells me, kissing Finn.

'Not as odd as it's been for me!'

I'm thinking: Simon went out into the real world again. After all that we went through together yesterday. The sound of Finn's wild heartbeat on the monitor, thundering like a train about to derail; the slow, eerie entrance Finn made, with his head to one side, carefully considering the first thing which met his gaze – the inside of my thigh – as if he were a camper emerging from a tent, taking his time to appraise the weather before pushing the rest of his body out. The sight of the umbilical cord, glorious in its violent colours, like something washed up on a beach, still pulsing with the salty green trace of the sea.

We'd glanced around the birthing room as we left and were stunned into silence by the devastation we'd managed to wreak: blood-splattered cloths, towels, sheets, paper and hospital gowns strewn everywhere. Like the scene of a violent attack.

After all that, Simon had bought shoes. He went out. He could be with his mates in a dark, rowdy place where he didn't have to worry about the effect of smoke on mini, pure lungs. He didn't feel ashamed of breasts ready to cascade milk at every baby squeak. While I had lain in bed, my hand on my belly, trying to persuade myself that no one was in there any more, that I was now only myself again, and not believing it; feeling my boundaries dissolve and waver, making me blur out of focus like a bad photograph; during all of that Simon had simply gone out and downed a pint of Guinness.

I narrow my eyes, watching Simon as he smiles into the baby's plastic crib. A sliver of resentment wedges between us.

Finn is sleeping now, his face sealed up, his mouth a closed purse. Hard to believe, looking at him in all his angelic rosiness, that he was up most of the night, fussing and screaming.

'His nose is like an eraser on the end of a pencil,' I say.

'He's gorgeous,' Simon responds.

Finn opens one eye. The other is crusted with sleep.

'How predictable you are,' Finn says.

The hospital ward holds its breath. The crockery on the tea trolley heading our way crashes to a halt. Simon blinks rapidly. I sit bolt upright, staring over at the crib. Last night I thought I'd imagined it, dreamed it, possibly. But Finn's voice is clear and steady. A lovely little voice, not babyish or wheedling. Trying out your handful of notes, I think. Plath again.

But then the metallic, clanking, hospital noises start up again. Cups of tea and KitKats trundle towards my bed. Curtains are swishily pulled; the other visitors continue talking. Simon is rustling in the plastic carrier, oblivious.

'When you said disposable knickers, I had a bit of a problem. I had to ask the assistant. It was hilarious,' he is saying.

*He didn't hear him.* Finn didn't speak. The pause was nothing, I realise. It's all in my head. Nothing has ground to a halt – everything hurtles on as normal. Simon is holding up a pack of Boots maternity knickers in size Large: 18–20.

'Size eighteen! I've never been a size eighteen in my life!'

'I didn't look, I just picked up the first packet she pointed out to me . . .'

'I know I've put weight on, but not *that* much!'

Simon laughs sheepishly, recognising that he's made a gaffe.

'Most men bring their wives flowers,' I say.

He thinks I'm joking. I turn the packet of paper knickers over in my hand, staring at the photo of a smiling blonde model, the supposedly new mother. Lying on his back in the crib, Finn opens both his eyes, his expression inscrutable. He opens his tiny triangle-shaped mouth, makes instead a perfect O. He looks just as if he is silently laughing.

'I think he needs a feed,' Simon suggests, tentatively picking him up. Finn's head wobbles alarmingly as Simon struggles to get the hold right, do it the way the midwife showed him, supporting the baby's head.

Simon is rocking his son, while I twitch with impatience.

'Give him to me, then,' I say greedily.

Finn is handed over. I brush his cheek with my nipple and my body stops its clamour. Simon sits creakily on the bed again; his hands fall on his lap, open.

The doctor comes to check the baby before we go. He sits on the bed in Simon's place and Simon stands up, watching while Dr Solenke rotates Finn's fat little legs in a gesture which looks cruel and unnatural. Finn raises his eyebrows in surprise but doesn't cry. The doctor gives his tiny testicles a quick squeeze. Finn flaps his arms vigorously.

Simon shifts from foot to foot.

'The thing is, Paula's quite keen to get out of here,' he says. 'Are you letting her out today, do you think? She hates hospitals.'

'As long as the baby's fine, I've no problem with that,'

says Dr Solenke, placing a finger into Finn's fist, which clasps it with an instinct both light and swift. A foxglove closing.

'Is there anything unusual about our baby?' I ask, leaning over to stare at Finn's wizened belly button, examine the blood hardening on the teeth of the white plastic clamp.

'No,' says Dr Solenke cheerily, handing the nappy and sleepsuit out to Simon to replace. The doctor smiles his grin for new parents. 'You have yourselves a cheeky little chappie.'

The phrase startles me, it's ridiculous. I shoot Finn a nervous glance, half expecting him to laugh again. Thankfully he's preoccupied, putting all his energy into resisting Simon's clumsy attempts to dress him. An exquisitely tender feeling comes over me as I watch Simon's big hand pulling the baby's limp arm through the sleeve of the sleepsuit. The doctor is finishing his form filling, distracted, glad to be able to tick us off, move to the next bed.

'Now's your chance,' I say to Finn. 'Speak now or forever hold your peace.' The doctor and Simon smile at me, as if I'm making a weak joke.

But Finn only stares up at me, keeps his mouth in a firm closed line, his lips pursed like two fat maggots.

So I discover that Finn only talks to me. It doesn't matter if we're alone or with others; whether the situation is noisy or silent. I can't control it or predict it and I can't get anyone else to hear it, either. I tell myself that no matter how powerful and genuine it sounds, it can only be my imagination. But this explanation just doesn't ring true. Finn's voice, his beautiful voice, low and clear and pure, is as unmistakable as the starlings on the roof of our bedroom.

All I have to do is keep my ears open.

Our first night at home with Finn we are in bed by nine o'clock. Simon has lit candles on the bedside table and brought the Moses basket up to our room, placed all the flowers we've been sent in vases on the floor around the bed; the room is filled with the scent of freesia and white roses. A cross between a church and a funeral parlour, with the baby in the centre, like an offering.

We sit in bed together, me feeding again, pyjama top falling open on breasts grown lumpy and enormous, threaded with veins like a Stilton cheese. Finn's intense sucking fills the silence, punctuated by breathing, hungry and desperate. I'm amazed at the ferocity of his need, his desire to suck, to keep sucking, to draw everything towards himself. *Food and drink you are to me*. It's what poets say about being in love, but when is it actually true? Only for babies. Falling in love seems remarkably similar to a newborn's desperate need for its mother. The thought makes me shudder.

'Do you feel differently about me? About my body?' I ask Simon.

'No, I don't,' he says.

A gallant response. He closes his book, tries to kiss my throat. Finding Finn's body somehow in the way, he kisses the baby's head instead.

'I feel differently about you,' I say.

'In what way?' Simon's voice is anxious. Surprised.

'I don't know. Just different,' I insist. I'm holding Finn up, burping him. Simon tries to snuggle up to me.

'What kind of different? Worse? Better?'

'Just different. I don't know.'

I get out of bed to lay Finn in his Moses basket, tuck his drowsy sleeping form under the blue Scottie-dog blanket I bought all those months ago, those months when I was trying to imagine my child, trying to imagine doing exactly this.

'He's all right, my dad,' Finn says. 'Don't give him a hard time.'

'Boys and fathers!' I reply. 'It's all idolisation, nothing real.'

'What?' Simon says. 'Of course it's real.'

I step around to Simon's side of the bed to blow out the candles, blowing so hard that wax splatters the wall behind.

'Candles. They're a bit stupid, aren't they, with a new baby around?'

Simon doesn't answer. His back is to me, to the centre of the bed. I want to snuggle up to his warmth now but the gesture freezes me out. I know I've hurt him and the thought gives me a twinge of satisfaction. He has no idea, I say to myself. He doesn't understand – me, us. Now it's *us*, for the first time. Someone with whom to share being misunderstood.

So we have an argument on the third day; a huge, savage argument, quite different from any we've had before.

I'm tempted to tell him. I'd really love to tell him, to shout it at him: 'Your baby talks and you don't even realise it! You're so *not in this relationship* that you can't even hear him! I'm different now, entirely different and you can't see it.'

I don't know what the row is about. Nothing. Everything. It starts with Simon suggesting that maybe it's not that helpful for me to pick up Finn every time he cries. The words 'rod for your own back' are not actually uttered, but manage to inveigle their way into the atmosphere anyway. I'm steaming, accusing Simon of being cold, cruel, unfeeling, of trying to control me, being a control freak, in fact – yes, that's it, a control freak – and now he wants to extend this Hitleresque attitude to our poor helpless baby, who after all is probably only hungry, for God's sake, and has Simon got a problem with that? And Simon after a bit of shouting back says no, he's sorry, what does he know. 'Fine,' he snaps. 'You do things your own way, only don't come crying to me when it doesn't work out, and if you want my help you should stop treating me like a moron, making me feel like an idiot. You should be glad I'm willing to help since plenty of men –'

'Aahhhhh! Now we are getting down to it! You think of it as *helping*. What you're saying is, Finn is primarily *my* responsibility and when you take care of him you're doing me some kind of *favour*.'

'No, no I didn't say that! But the reality is – you've got the breasts, the *equipment*, you're what he wants –'

'So you're jealous, is that it?'

'Not jealous, but I do feel left out, yes! Because you're not letting me in.'

I suppose there's some truth in this. I don't want to let him in. I keep thinking: Nothing has changed for him. And everything has changed for me. *Love divides the lovers.* Poetry again. Reading it is like scattering spores – you've no idea where the words might land, where or when or if they'll take seed. I remember not understanding that line when I read it, but now it pops into my head and sticks there, indelible.

We are still going for it hammer and tongs when the midwife arrives for her morning visit. Simon lets her in. She's small, Irish, with a beaky nose and the smallest feet I've ever seen on a grown woman. That and the flattest of chests. I haven't dared ask but I'm pretty sure she's never had a baby herself.

Simon goes to make her a cup of tea.

'Can I ask you something?' I venture, while he is out of the room.

She's opening her bag, getting out the scales and looking

around our cramped flat for a space on the floor to put them on.

'Of course,' she says, without looking up.

'I read somewhere that babies can see sounds or hear colours. That their senses can get mixed up, you know. It's a sort of miswiring in their brain or something. A bit like poetry, when images suggest themselves for sounds.'

When she doesn't reply, I prompt: 'Is that true?'

'When I said "of course" I was thinking cradle cap. Jaundice. Sore nipples. That kind of thing.'

'Oh. I see.'

A pause.

'Well, I have another question. Sometimes when I look at him, I think he is talking to me. That I can hear him talking. I don't know if it's my imagination, or some miswiring in *my* brain, making me hear things, the way a schizophrenic does. Or hearing things when I should just be imagining them or seeing them.'

She leans over the Moses basket to unpeel a sleeping Finn from his swaddle of blankets.

'You're a gorgeous little fella then, aren't you?' she says.

'Do any other women, have you heard of any women who tell you that their baby – that they hear their baby talk to them?'

'Oh yes.' The midwife, Frances, her name is, is unwrapping him down to his nappy. My question doesn't faze her at all. Her bony fingers leave white marks on Finn's naked chest, as she holds him above the scales. 'The first few days with a new baby, plenty of women tell me some pretty odd things.'

She tears off pieces from a huge roll of green scratchy paper, lining the scales before placing Finn's naked body on them. He lies very still, waiting for the rest of her reply.

The clink of cups tells me that Simon is standing in the doorway.

'What a big boy! Three point four kilos, isn't that grand?' Frances says, noting the result in her notebook and smiling with satisfaction at Finn.

'Your hands are freezing!' Finn says.

I glance from Frances to Simon to Finn. It's obvious no one else heard him. He's screaming his head off now, protesting at being dressed, so Frances hands him to Simon while she nudges me towards the bathroom to check my stitches and talk 'women's stuff'.

'No need for your husband to be there for that, now is there?' she says, leading the way. She gives me a showy wink. 'Retain some of the mystery, now isn't that true?'

'Mystery! You've got to be kidding. He was at the birth, for God's sake,' Finn shouts from the other room. Frances ignores him, closes the bathroom door.

Frances sits herself down on the closed toilet seat. I get the impression she's used to working in homes with rather more space than ours, but she's improvising admirably.

'Now,' she says. 'Do you want to tell me what's the matter?'

'Nothing's the matter,' I reply, like a sulky child.

She crosses one leg over the other. Her shoes are dark with laces. The smallness of her feet, the neatness of her legs in their dark tights fills me with sadness.

'I used to be neat and small,' I say.

She squints at me, eyebrows drawn into a sharp frown.

'I'm someone who really needs her sleep,' I tell her. 'That's all.'

'Ah, *sleepless nights*. Counts for a lot, to be sure. No wonder the Chinese used it as a form of torture, now, eh!'

'I think I'm in the Twilight Zone. Everyone else is in bed and sleeping and I've somehow become part of the animal kingdom, with a hot snuggling creature suckling at me like a piglet. And Simon's just lying there snoring.'

Her frown re-emerges. 'I've brought my *Post-Natal*

*Depression Checklist* and I'll not go until I've been through it with you.' She folds her arms across her flat chest.

I decide to sit on the edge of the bath and as I'm about to lower myself down, Frances leaps up.

'What am I thinking of? You must sit down – not there, that'll do your stitches no good at all.'

She gives up her seat on the loo and I take her place. Simon knocks on the door. 'Do you want your tea in there, you two?'

'Give us a little while,' Frances says, taking the lid off her pen.

We go through the whole checklist and I score twenty-five out of a possible thirty. But none of the questions concern babies who talk, the way Finn does, or women who feel their boundaries have become hazy or who are scared to look up at the bathroom mirror, in case they find that they have no reflection and they really have entered the Twilight Zone.

My mother arrives on the fifth day, when Simon has to go back to work. She tidies up, hoovers, brings me two extra vases from the Oxfam shop. Says nothing about the vases around the bed in our room, although the positioning does look somehow dubious to me now; a little too reverential. She discards the flowers which have turned crunchy and brown and replaces them with ones from a bunch of daffodils she's brought from her garden.

I stand watching in the doorway to the kitchen, holding Finn in my arms, still in my dressing-gown. Finn is watching too, both eyes open. I'm thinking that his eyes are the exact colour and shape of miniature mussel shells. I'm looking at him, not at her, so I'm surprised when she says softly, 'He looks like you did as a baby.'

I glance up to find she's right beside us. She brushes Finn's cheek.

'You had a dimple just there. And you were so happy, always smiling and gurgling. Hardly cried at all.'

This is a new version of myself. I know I was an awkward, terrified child with a fear of parties, an imaginary friend and all kinds of other eccentricities; and a red-hot teenager, flaming with acne and feminist politics, so the picture of myself as a contented, dimpled baby is a revelation.

Now Mum is emptying the contents of the linen basket on to the kitchen floor so that she can throw everything in the wash. She has never been allowed so close to our underwear before and I can feel her satisfaction at getting her hands on Simon's boxer shorts and socks and Finn's little white vests with their ribbon ties at the front. Belatedly I'm grateful for the disposable knickers.

'So there was nothing . . . odd about me as a baby?' I ask her, while her guard is down, her back to me, pouring powder into the drawer of the washing machine.

'You were an odd child,' she says breezily.

'I know that. But was I an odd baby? Did you like me?'

'These forty-degree washes. How can they expect you to get a white bib clean on that?' she mutters.

'She's stalling,' Finn says. 'You know she never liked you.'

It's true that my relationship with my mother has never been an easy one. I always had the sense that she wished I was someone else. Someone who found life more straightforward. Who didn't live so much with her skin unpeeled.

'You were a lovely baby,' Mum says firmly, closing the drawer with a click and a small splash. 'Shall we go next door and watch *Neighbours*?'

We settle in front of the telly, safe ground, I know, since it prevents conversation. I hand the baby to Mum, lowering myself awkwardly into my chair and then watch surreptitiously, jealously, as she cradles him, coos to him.

100

I'm waiting to hear what he'll say, hear what he thinks of her, but under the spell of her determined rocking he soon falls asleep.

'You were a fast delivery!' Mum says, unprompted. 'You shot out of me. The midwife practically had to catch you, like a slippery fish that might have wanted to slip right back, over the side of the boat! I remember it like it was yesterday. It was October and the middle of a lightning storm. Trust you to pick an occasion like that to make your entrance. Sometimes a purple light flashed in the living-room window – I was at home, you know – so that you really did look silver, or at least a funny pale blue colour, and a fish is exactly what came to mind. But a fish with the most perfect, tiniest rose-pink mouth. I took one look at you and knew you'd be – unusual. Fragile.'

'Trouble, you mean.'

'*Fragile*. That's what I said. Like I could never relax about you. Always worrying.'

'You didn't have to worry. You took it on yourself to worry!'

'You'll see,' is all she says. Eyeing me carefully as she says this, behind her glasses. Finn sleeps blissfully in her arms.

The curse of the Bad Fairy at Sleeping Beauty's christening. *You will feel enormous pain, now you are a mother*. Great. Thanks a bunch.

'Great,' I say. 'And now the good news?'

For the good news, she nods towards Finn; sleeping with one hand resting on his blanket, the fingers spread, like a tiny starfish.

As she leaves, my mum says, stiffly, with some effort: 'You probably think I got everything wrong.'

'No, I don't. I don't think that.'

'You do,' Finn says.

She roots in her bag for her umbrella, gives me a quick

101

kiss on the cheek. She smells of face powder, of almonds and old-fashioned lily of the valley perfume and all the things she always smelled of, all through my childhood.

'We all do our best, that's all we can do. But you were a gorgeous baby. It was impossible not to love you.'

The door's closed and she's halfway down the drive before I hear it properly. It's the most she's ever said. The closest she's come. It feels like an admission. *I wanted not to love you, but I did, in spite of myself.* Isn't that what I've felt from her, all my life? I know the circumstances of my birth, my father's death just before it, I know she must have resented me. I suppose I should be grateful or cheered up or something, because wasn't I asking her, wasn't that what I wanted to know?

Where did I come from, how did I get here? Why am I here?

*Love set you going, like a fat gold watch*

Sometimes even poetry lets you down. *I don't know, I don't know, no one knows.* That's more like it.

That night Simon brings champagne, fish and chips, a baby magazine. I'm lying in the bath, something I've waited to do all day; the highlight of my day, when the baby sleeps and I can get a half-hour to myself.

'I can't drink champagne when I'm breast-feeding,' I tell him, when he shows me the bottle. His face falls.

'My life will never be the same again,' I say, and burst into tears.

He sits on the edge of the bath, stroking my hair. He never knows what to do when I cry, but at least he doesn't tell me to stop crying or croon, 'Never mind,' or any other such crap. After a while I stop and stare up at him, suddenly tearless and spiteful.

'I feel like I hate you. And Mum. I hate everyone except Finn.'

'Well, it's good that you don't hate Finn, I suppose.'

'I didn't know it would be like this. Maybe I *am* depressed. The baby keeps talking to me. I can hear his comments on every subject, and it's never favourable. He hates everyone as well. Oh, that's not true, I suppose. He likes you.'

So I've told Simon without any fanfare and now I'm searching his face to see what he makes of it.

'Well, he's told me he loves you,' Simon says quietly, struggling with the champagne cork.

Twisting around in the bath, I cause a great wave of water to slop over the side. The cork pops.

'He doesn't speak to you! He only talks to me. Only *I* can hear him.'

I'm adamant about this. Simon is avoiding my gaze. From the tension in his jaw, his shoulders, I pick up great trepidation, nervousness. I know he is afraid for me. Then, with some effort, he looks up. Holds out the bath towel. I let him wrap me in it, feel his arms envelop me, just as if I was a small child. Rain patters on the windows outside. From the bedroom I hear Finn begin crying, clawing sounds, like a cat scraping at a door.

Simon makes a move to go to him but turns to say, 'If you shut me out, Paula, things won't get any better. I want to help you. And I want to take care of our child.'

'You think I'm mad then?'

'No . . .'

Finn's yelling gets louder, harder to ignore. Simon hands me a half-filled mug of champagne, which I stare into, as if it were a wishing well.

'You don't really think Finn talks, then? You didn't really hear him say he loves me?'

'I don't know. I suppose not.'

'You know, Doctor, you should never enter into the delusions of your clients. It doesn't help them and it's not honest.'

He smiles. A big broad smile. 'But it's so obvious he loves you. No collusion necessary.'

'So you're not going to have me locked up then?'

'No.'

Finn yells from down the corridor, 'Get over here! Stop talking to each other and think about me for a change!'

Still wrapped in the towel I pad to the baby room. I fumble for the light. The room smells of something sharp and piquant – new paint, lemon sherberts, a new presence. Finn's world. I'm scared of it. The world of milk teeth wrapped in cotton wool. Snippets of baby hair, drawings of stick people. Keepsakes, loss. The terrifying thought occurs to me that I've never loved anyone this much and a newborn seems too small to bear that burden.

Finn is in his Moses basket, thrashing his arms and legs in fury as I approach. His blankets are kicked off and the room is a little chilly, a boat mobile dangling eerily above his bed. Rain splashes my skin as I close his bedroom window.

He stops crying as soon as I pick him up.

'About time,' he grumbles. 'Where've you been? Didn't you hear me? I've been yelling for ages.'

'Sssh now, I'm here . . .'

Here's someone, a whole new person to learn about. Someone who didn't exist a week ago. He seems to be looking at me, opening his eyes a little wider than he was capable of only a day or two ago. It's disquieting to be scrutinised so closely.

'I'm Paula. Your mother,' I tell him.

A long pause. I feel something more needs to be said.

'I hope you don't feel you drew a short straw.'

Wind and rain lash the fine membrane of the house. Finn gazes up at me with his glittering fish-shaped eyes and, tactfully, says nothing.

# Mala's Baby
## *Chandani Lokugé*

Priya turned again on the mat, and this time twisted himself into a tangle of bones. He turned yet again, then lifted himself up on his elbow. Mala's baby lay just a little distance away. He knew it was hungry – but it was always hungry. He could hear it suck on air, as it lay naked on its threadbare cloth. Its arms and legs would be flaying weakly, sticking out of the shell of its body. He stretched out an arm and tapped the fragile ribcage until he felt it lull, the limbs slowly relaxing, the sucking fading into fitful sleep. Leaning further, he felt for the tiny fingers that would grasp his if they could.

He knew it was very, very late. It was that time of night, when even the sound of the sea was subdued by the blanketing darkness. He peered around the room. The small wick burned before the picture of Mary and the Baby Jesus. It flickered bravely on the dregs of oil in the red glass bowl. Shadows played on the picture, and small points of light sparkled in the eyes of Baby Jesus. Priya's thoughts wandered away to a dream, constantly dreamt – of Mala's baby transforming into the chubby little Jesus smiling into Mary's face. And Mala, if only Mala, like Mary in the picture, could suddenly gaze down at him in the gloom of this room. If only. He curled up on the chill mat, and seemed to hear Mala mutter in her sleep and cuddle him anyway. But there was no Mala. It was on such a night, months ago, that their father had chased her out of the house. Any night, if Priya listened, he would hear her sobs. They were everywhere; sometimes, like tonight, they were so close he could almost touch them. At other times, he didn't know which were his sobs, and which were hers. When the wind was high, they whimpered and curled into homeless corners.

Even as he tried to shut out the dream of her, he heard a gentle knock on the wooden door. He half sat up and then lay back. It was the wind, playing tricks on his foolish fancies, as his mother would admonish sharply, if he were to call to her. But there it was again. He crept up on his hands and knees so as not to awaken the sleeping baby or his mother lying on the other side, and listened with his ear to the door. Then, like a streak of lightning, he was on his feet pulling down the wooden slat that locked it. And there, in the light of the slight crescent moon, was Mala.

'*Amme*, *amme*, our Mala is here,' he yelled back into the house, but his voice, a high treble, was no more than a squeak.

'Mala *akka* has come home,' he whispered. He caught hold of her skirt and pulled. But there was no need; there was hardly any resistance. She entered the house. It was as if the wind had gathered force to blow her, like a defence-less leaf, into the room.

Quickly he closed the door on the night.

He twisted his arms around her waist then and buried his face in her dress. She held him to her, stroking his back and crooning. He pressed himself closer and closer, touching and feeling her, and then drew back violently. He gazed at her in horror. The hardness of her stomach was unmistakable. Had he not felt it each time his mother was having a younger sister? He shivered. He looked up at her beseechingly. Why, Mala, why again? Didn't she remember how it had been the last time? But he said nothing, and together they looked towards their mother who stirred on her mat and muttered.

And when she sat up like she'd seen a ghost, and moaned, 'Mala?' they drew closer to her. Priya knew she had been waiting for this. Every night she moaned Mala's name in her sleep. But if he dared mention it in the daytime, she would yell at him, 'If she comes within sight of this house, I'll cut her up and throw her in the sea,' but she'd look back furtively in the direction of the road. Like him, she searched the distance for the speck of red that could be Mala's skirt.

Now Priya switched on the light. Shadows that crouched all over the floor during his long vigils fled to corners. Mala, there was only Mala. Priya was never to forget it – the way the light from the naked bulb circled her in the centre of the room, and the warmth that radiated from her to enfold him. But she did not smile, or pull him to her. She only looked around sullenly.

'Your father's gone to sea,' their mother said, just as sullenly. Now that she knows that Mala is alive, she's going to nag her, Priya thought, full of resentment. He drew closer to his sister.

'Go and make us some tea, *malli*,' Mala said to him, barely looking in his direction. And uncertainly, he moved backwards towards the kitchen. But he kept looking back into the living room. He couldn't bear to be away – perhaps she'd disappear again.

He stood at the doorway, until the water boiled. She was bent over her baby, her face gaunt and sad. Suddenly, closing the distance, she gathered it in her arms. She began to kiss him and feel his rickety body. He saw her, more beautiful than the picture of Mother Mary up there in the crevice in the wall. The next day, after all this was over, he would squat on the wet sand, and sketch his sister's face gazing down at her baby. And, as a wave erased it, he would stare far, far into the distance. Then, kneeling just there on the sand, palms clasped, he would pray to the gods who controlled their lives.

'Take that cursed child where you are going, don't leave him behind for us,' his mother said in a cruel voice. Priya cringed from the change in his sister's face.

'*Aney, amme,* do keep quiet,' he pleaded.

When Priya returned with the tea, Mala and his mother were sitting side by side on the floor, leaning against the wall. His mother was stroking Mala's hair, trying to discipline the long wavy tresses, in the old familiar way. It seemed to Priya that his sister had never gone away. He gave them their glasses of tea and, holding the sugar-bottle under his arm, scraped half spoons into their palms. He had also prepared a bottle of plain tea for the baby that he now held to its lips. Mala watched, licking the sugar from her palm between sips of tea. She did not offer to feed the baby. Soon the little sucking lips fell apart, and the baby slept tiredly, its hunger momentarily appeased. As Priya gave Mala the half-empty bottle, he saw her rub her eyes. He was happy to see her cry. It seemed to him that she would melt that way, into tears, and then she would be the old Mala again, dimpling and laughing, and with sidelong glances, flirting with all the young men. How she was changed.

'Go to sleep, *malli* – come here, lie against me.' Mala spoke to him at last in the voice he remembered, and happily Priya crawled up to her to lay his head on her lap. As in the old days, he felt her fingers absently ruffling his hair.

'How are the younger sisters?' Mala asked their mother.

'The good Sisters have found them two houses after they saw what happened to you. They don't get paid much, but they are fed, I think. I go and visit them sometimes,' she replied.

'That's good,' Mala murmured. And then, 'You haven't grown at all, you sprat,' she said, bending over her brother.

'How can he? When that unfortunate half-caste of yours drinks up all the money in the house?' their mother snapped back.

Mala leaned tiredly against the wall. And as she stretched back, their mother suddenly noticed the protrusion of her stomach outlined against her dress. And she threw up her arms.

'Mala, again! Oh, you are cursed and so are we. Oh, Mother of God, let the sea take us all, and spare us the shame.'

'Just let me rest awhile, *amme*, I am so tired. So very tired,' Mala sighed.

'Let her be, will you, *amme*? Please don't scold her,' Priya said.

'You keep quiet. Who was it this time? Whose child is that now?' his mother asked.

Priya wanted only to close his ears against the shame and fury in his mother's voice. But there was no shutting it out. And there was the sag of his sister's body, as she remembered it all.

'The master of the big house,' she said in a monotone. 'That's where I've been living after going away from here. The lady was kind, but I had to leave.'

A long, lonely silence followed. Outside, the wind had changed. It rose and rose, and shrieked and howled as if it hungered for them all. They heard the coconut palms tear out of the trees and swing down to the ground. Priya thought how he would have to drag them to the back of the house tomorrow, so his mother could weave them for the Sunday Fair. Since Mala and his two younger sisters had gone away, they had extra work to do, all except their father who sailed away to sea every evening, drank toddy every night, and slept it all away in the morning.

Mala sighed heavily. 'Men are like animals when they're drunk,' she said. How like his mother's voice was his sister's. Priya had not noticed it before. 'They're all the same. If the child lives, and it's a girl, I will call her Kumari. They had a daughter at the big house, and that was her name. She's dead now.'

The silence fell on them again. It stretched and stretched. Priya lay against Mala. He felt that someone had knifed them all a second time. How could they stop the bleeding again and again? He had no idea who had done it, whether it was his mother or his father or his sister, or the master of the big house, or the babygrowing in Mala. What he knew was that one morning he would open the front door to find this next baby on their doorstep, just like the first time.

There would be a big uproar. His mother would tear her hair and beat her breasts, flinging curses on Mala and on the unknown father of the infant, and his father would rush up and down the beach with the fish-knife, flinging it around and slashing imaginary people, the stale smell of toddy and of the sea spewing from his breath. All the neighbouring old women would gather around the house in twos and threes gossiping about Mala and her way-wardness. They'd remember how she sauntered past their houses enticing their sons to follow her. They'd remember how she'd run back from the sea after a bath, her hair glistening in the evening sun, her breasts half-revealed by the thin bath cloth. And they'd say she deserved what she got . . . And it would be left to Priya to take the baby in his arms, carry it to the bench behind the house and skulk there with it, until it was safe to slink back in. The only difference this time would be that the baby would have a name. And Mala would be sixteen years old, instead of fifteen.

Another baby, he thought, another mouth to feed. He could see his mother stand up on the stool reaching for the broken-handled cup that she kept hidden behind the picture of Mary and Jesus. Desperately, she'd circle its emptiness with her fingers, and then turn it upside down, as if it would magically spill a shower of coins on them. Then she'd place the cup back, clasp her palms and mutter a prayer to the picture. At last, she'd turn and say to him: 'Mother Mary will look after us.'

But Priya knew better. He'd just have to work twice as hard to contribute to the broken-handled cup. He would return to the cabana at the far end of the beach and go with the rich white man. Mala had gone to the far end of the beach too. That was what had happened the first time. And that was why the baby was a funny light shade with no-colour eyes. And that's why everyone called it Mala's *paraya*. Still hurting, he turned his face towards her body, breathing in her smell, her sweat, her cushioning warmth. And then, as if in a dream that only they could share, he felt her hand gently guiding his palm to the side of her stomach. And ever so softly, against her quivering skin, he could feel the tap tap of the unborn child. Again and again he felt it, and he knew that through him, his sister listened to it too, the fluttering life of the little one.

'If the lady is kind, leave the child at their doorstep, Mala. That's all there is to do. Don't dump it here – your father will kill it.' The mother's voice had shifted to the passivity that often followed a violent row with their father.

Priya closed his eyes and ears. He only wished that he was older so he could have his own place where his sister could have her baby. He began to suck on the knuckle of his thumb. Only eleven and good for nothing, as his mother said.

'. . . don't sew up the mouth of the pillowcase, now,' he heard his mother say to Mala between sleep and dream. 'That bodes ill for the mother,' and '. . . in the last months, remember to throw some paddy on the ground, and bend down to pick up the grains one at a time. That way, you won't have too much labour pain. I remember . . .' His sister murmured something in reply. Where would she have the money for pillows and paddy? Their voices dripped with sleepless anguish.

And he heard Mala say, perhaps sometime later, '*Aney, amme*, what is going to happen to me? It was very bad the first time, all alone at the hospital so far away. The attendants are cruel women . . . I hoped the child would die.'

And again, 'They will not help me at the big house, *amme*. The master didn't even come downstairs when I left. Can't I stay here, at home?'

Much later, he awakened fully. He half sat up. His sister lay fast asleep with her head on their mother's shoulder. And the mother sat very straight, the baby in her lap, staring straight at the picture of Mary and Jesus.

'Are you praying, *amme*?' he asked timidly.

'No,' she said, without removing her eyes from the picture. 'Your father will be home in an hour or so. It's nearly light. Will you make more tea, so your sister can have some before she leaves.'

'Is she leaving?' he asked, dismayed. His mother turned now to cuff him over his ears.

'Must you always ask questions?' she said, but there was no anger in her voice, just that rough and fleeting tenderness that Priya knew so well. They all lived for such moments, but today he was not warmed by it. Her words fell like pebbles into a deep dark well.

The tears springing to his eyes, he wandered away to the kitchen. He opened the window and peered out through the poles. The wind was down, and it was going to be a clear day. In the faint light of dawn, he could see the backyard strewn with last night's storm.

Soon they would spot their father's catamaran heading home and his mother would call to him to go down by the beach to help haul it in. He hoped it would be a good catch this morning.

# The 'Kursk'

## *Eva Sallis*

A Russian submarine hit a mine from World War Two and fell down into the dark cold silence of the Norwegian Sea.

The computer graphics recreating the scene make the water an even aqua. The submarine looks like an oblong egg, with five stylised men in the cutaway cross-section representing the 118 who are on board. Cartoon flame flares and then fades as the sub dives. A black star appears on the side when it lies broken on the cyan-yellow seafloor. I flick to another channel to see the mine and the egg collide with a fateful flare and then the same scene in aqua. Then the surface of the Norwegian Sea appears on the screen – cuts of pitching ships, slags of grey and murky seas, men in yellow struggling on slick decks, rain-drenched warships standing by, then dead hulks of cracked and deserted submarines in Murmansk Harbour; and then, the *US Alaska*, a trim uniform grey in a sunny Persian Gulf.

I watch television news to pass the time. The great weight of my body presses me into the sofa and I feel my belly wince.

I am bored with this baby who can squirm in fluid athletic arcs, a playful cat rolling; who can make my belly square. Can press his heel into the inside of my ribcage and stretch. Can headbutt me from the solar plexus, straining to see out through the veil of red that is me. I'm bored with looking inward to a belly world. He sleeps and wakes when he wishes and knows which bits to kick to make me jump. He can stretch out a small hand in wonder and touch the inside of my skin when it glows with the orange point of light from a penlight torch, and I'm bored with that, too.

This is what I see reflected tonight in the window behind the television: the spindly legs and arms and head are me and in the middle is the impossible, taut moon, a baby sphere, carried awkwardly, shocking.

I want him out of me, out of water and into the air.

After the news of the submarine, I dreamed I was Baba Yaga's hut, top-heavy on plucked chicken legs. I scampered away from Baba Yaga, but she caught me, scaled up a leg and gave me a walloping from within. She bolted the door to my body and drew the curtains, and I trudged away with her inside me.

This morning the rescue operations have begun. The survivors in the submarine have tapped out their messages; the Americans, Norwegians and Russians have haggled, weighing secrets against lives; and the Russians are preparing for the laborious extraction. They have to succeed. My throat hurts, my muscles tighten and the baby inside me rolls and pitches.

I can hear their voices, warming the darkness, singing a Russian folksong. Men's voices, and the harder timbre of boys. They are huddled together as one under the hatch that they cannot open.

The midwives say that he is engaged posterior but that this is nothing to worry about.

I'm tired of advice and advice-givers. I see their sideways glances and the way they angle through a crowd to sit next to me. They visit with presents so I can't throw them out. They appear behind the eyes of my friends and relatives.

'Don't put him down on his back. Or is it his belly? One of them can be fatal. I knew a girl . . .'

'Sing to him *in utero*. He can hear, you know . . .'

'Don't let them bully you . . . It's the best thing for him, but if you let them bully you . . . I know you can breast-feed – it's just not easy at first. Don't let them pressure you. It's all natural anyway. When I had mine . . .'

'Have you been to classes? They are so much fun. No? You *should*. You can share the experience with others who *understand*.'

I am sick of picking fights with everyone, of hitting back first and making sure no one feels safe to come up and touch me. They come, fingers wriggling and outstretched towards my belly, head on one side, shoulders hunched, eyes squinting, mouth smiling and guttering with self-diminishing syllables containing lots of 'g's. But I'm tired of feeling as though I have to fight.

I am tired of their sweet and sour birth stories. I am tired of gentle, sweetened malice.

The Australians have a bathysphere bigger and better than anyone else's, but it will take a day and a night and a day to airlift and ship through the storm to the site. The Australians are smug – the Russians haven't asked, in any case. The Americans run stories on how crap the Russian sub fleet is, more pictures of the rusted shells in Murmansk, more acrimony. Everyone says that if they weren't hiding something, they'd have asked the Americans. The Russians ask the Norwegians who say it can't be done in this weather. More slurried decks and slick yellow coats. The English send a bathysphere so small that only one load of men will be lifted from their 'watery grave', and only if it can dock. The world snorts in disapproval and someone writes on the CNN website: '*To any Russians who are reading this: most Americans feel for you and pray for your loved ones.*'

I see them in my dreams. They have finished with songs and folktales, stories and commands. They have broken apart in the darkness, fighting and afraid. Then I hear the sweet percussion of the rescuers ringing into the airless cold. They cheer and laugh like small boys. They hug each other close and warm up again, and I smell their stale breath. But I am shaking with horror as my body grips me closer. I have already seen the late-night news: the careening bathysphere in the murky water; the shadowy hull at the wrong angle; and the repeated approach and retreat.

This morning, in the slo-mo computer graphics, the ungainly bubble cannot dock. Orange arrows make clear the current and the awkward angle of the hatch. But there is still hope in the 'race against time' and my heart is pounding. Today the storm is clearing and the current lessening, and surely tomorrow the craft will dock.

He has been tapping out his faint signals, telling me all is well in his red world and that the tide is turning. He has been kicking me for the adrenalin and begging for more sugar. He is hanging like a fruit bat, head downward, waiting for nightfall. I tell him he'll see a sharp white moon washing all the red world away.

'Has he kicked as often today?'

He is late and I am being battered by the world news and the short silences of the midwives.

The men in the submarine save their breath and I feel like screaming as I watch the news. They don't sing any more. I can hear a lone pen scratching in the dark and I can hear breathing. I can smell the unfrozen urine, the faeces, and their fear and disbelief.

It is time. I am out at sea, heaving between the waves of pain, waiting, angling to face the next. Each wave must be cleft with the smooth deep V of my breastbone at the right

117

angle, my head calm and still. A little to the left and a little to the right is turmoil and I'll go under. Heavy breath seems to drag at spent oxygen in the dark and cold. On and on, over and over I wait, then slide through pain. He stays remote, struggling on his own. I am weeping with the effort. It will take me a day and a night and a day to get there.

I am weeping for the submariners. How will they leave the dark cold silence? How long can their food last? How long can the oxygen be drawn in and out and in again? How long before the divers tear through the hatches and, with a flood, release them? I will them to break out. I can see them in their bright wetsuits, rising to the surface on one burbling thread of silver breath.

The midwife tells me that the hatches are damaged and cannot be opened. I see the bathysphere, useless and silly on its spindly legs, whimpering, hovering helplessly against the dark orb of a now silent sub.

I am dreaming now, no longer swimming, and my son's heart labours for me through each new storm. I am calm, as they say drowning men are. I am dreaming and all is bright and warm, and the voices and instruments clink and chitter about me. The midwives have left me to the sharp lights, voices and the scalpel. The voices tell me they have to go down into the vast oceans of my pain, down to the red world and cut him free, for his blood-oxygen is falling.

The television hangs above the barouche and crib, flickering. Covered heads. Tears on faces at Murmansk Harbour. Ungloved hands throw flowers into a calm green sea. And beside me, the pristine, angelic baby sleeps off his long journey, his face smooth, his breathing new but easy.

They will never see their sons again. I can't stop crying, looking down at mine.

# Look, You Can See Her Eyes

## *Margo Daly*

You were the ultimate souvenir, red-wrapped, hidden deep, brought secretly through Customs and Immigration. At this stage you could be likened to a parasite, or pollen, or a seed which fell from a bird's mouth: the most natural of migrations. I carried you through our country's welcome, pesticide spray in the aeroplane cabin. This was nothing compared to the cloud of pollution hanging over Cairo: a combination of straw-burning by rice farmers, smoke from potters' kilns and rubbish piles, exhaust fumes equivalent to smoking a pack of cigarettes a day. I dodged traffic with my eyes closed, clinging to Ali as cars ran through the red lights, a futile policeman waving a baton.

Your bags were already packed, little stowaway, while headlines told of the newest flood of boat people to Australia, from the Middle East, and you had already quickened inside me, and were kicking hard, as I watched the TV news of the same people escaping the crude detention camps deep in the continent's interior. I scanned heartbroken and angry Arab faces for clues to your hidden face. I imagined all they had dreamt Australia to be – skyscrapers and beaches, clean streets and modern homes – as you somersaulted inside me. Once I saw a dirty, dishevelled boy lying flat on his back on the busy pavement of Sharia Tahir. Ali and I were trying to get married. We thought it would be romantic to get married in Cairo, spent months obtaining pieces of paper, searching for witnesses. The sun beat down on the boy's face; it seemed he must be dead. I wanted to stop and see if he was OK. Ali said someone else would. I wanted to buy him some fruit, maybe a bunch of bananas, from the Bab al-Luq market. If he was not dead, only exhausted, he would wake up and eat. A gift while he was sleeping. But we didn't have time: we were trying to get married.

You were already there in Cairo, when all I wanted was a deep and profound sleep in the wintry afternoon light flowing through the balcony doors of our Heliopolis apartment. You were there on the overnight train to Luxor, on our honeymoon, increasing my bloodflow, so my nose suddenly flooded scarlet. Ali didn't offer his sympathy: sufferings had to be met stoically. After all, he had been trained since childhood to withstand thirst and hunger, even through the worst Ramadans, which fell in the long hot days of summer. A dry mouth could be rinsed with water, but not a single drop swallowed. You were with us in Alexandria, the day before Ramadan, when we drank hibiscus tea, *karkaday*, at a café in the souk, observing the feverish shopping activity and the men dextrously stretching and frying dough for rich and chewy cakes to break tomorrow's fast.

In the morning Ali and I caught the train back to Cairo, through the fertile delta of the Nile Valley. I discreetly sipped water from a plastic bottle, rustling quietly in my bag for the dried apricots and almonds bought to sustain me through the day. Although travellers were allowed to eat and drink, I saw no signs of consumption. You had to make up the fast some other time anyway: travelling was not an easy way out, Ali explained.

That night I was flying to Sydney. Ali would buy Eid presents for his family tomorrow – he laughed that my presence, a Westerner, forced the prices higher – and then take his flight to Dar El Baida: Casablanca. Modelled on Marseilles, it was Morocco's most modern city. He'd been to university, studied languages there. He would journey by bus to the small town where his family lived, surrounded by the now-greened winter hills of the Middle Atlas.

The embassy in Cairo advised that Ali's visa would take at least two months. He wanted to spend Ramadan with his family one last time, without me: it would be too difficult for me, too boring, everyone fasting, the streets deserted and quiet. But this would be a winter Ramadan of short cool days, easy to fast through, if I wanted. And he'd described Ramadan as the best time of the year. The long festive evenings, starting with the *fitr*: bowls of *harira*, with sweet chewy *chebbekia* and the best-quality dates. Later, the streets and cafés alive with people and music. The final celebration, Eid el Fitr, presents of new clothes, clean and fresh for another year. I longed to share it with him, to see his family again, but he pushed for me to go home. 'For your *own* celebration, Christmas,' he stressed. 'To be with your *own* family.'

'We won't be together for the new millennium,' I pleaded. 'We'll start the century apart.' Ali joked that we lived in different centuries, anyway; it was only the year 1420 by the Islamic calendar. When he saw my tears, he grabbed my left hand. 'We've made sacred vows,' he said, his eyes suddenly wet. So I was to go to Sydney and set up house, and when the visa arrived, he would come. '*In-shallah*,' he added. God willing.

My Kuwait Air flight coincided with dusk and a food tray loaded with *fitr* goodies. I looked at the fading city lights below. Ali would be at a café offering a free feast; for one night, without wife or family, he'd be seeking Muslim charity. Instead of fasting, the rich could feed others to attain grace. It didn't seem fair, I'd said. They should feed *and* fast. 'You always have an opinion,' Ali said, 'about everything.'

In Singapore, I transferred to a Qantas flight to Sydney. I chatted to the young freckled Australian beside me. It felt almost improper, after all these months, talking to a man I didn't know. With that intimacy of strangers, I told him how I'd met Ali in Bangkok five months before, travelled to meet his family in Morocco and married him in Cairo. My new friend wanted to ask his girlfriend to marry him on New Year's Eve. I waved my wedding band around and said it was the best thing he could do. 'It feels different being married. Totally different.' Safe and secure and loved.

Below, the world turned.

You were the one who was safe and secure, travelling unannounced.

My first days in Sydney are spent by the beach. My tiredness I equate with jetlag. What a parade of flesh is revealed to me! Unbelievable. The freedom of women. Unbelievable! The bars with tables looking on to the street, the women drinking and drunk! Unashamed. After three days, the faint revulsion for my own culture lifts: I daringly put on a short skirt, feeling the warm air on my legs as I do errands in the city. No men following me, no one staring. In my head I repeat, *Thank God I am a Western woman, thank God*. Resting in Hyde Park, I notice a couple entwined and kissing. In the park in Heliopolis, boys and girls, men and woman, sat chatting, but always apart. Once Ali lay on the grass and I leaned over him to laugh and tease, careful not to touch him. A man came from nowhere and waved at us in an agitated manner. '*Kein mushkill*,' he said. There's a problem. Ali sat up and I sprang away. '*Malish*,' he responded, turning on a charming smile. Never mind.

122

Soon, when Ali comes, we will be so free, I can almost feel the weight of his arm over my shoulder. Freedom. Unbelievable!

I cook my sister Cilla *chachouka* for dinner, a simple meal, one of Ali's favourites. It makes me feel closer to him. I simmer the tomatoes and onions and green pepper in olive oil until they are very tender, add cummin and paprika and then stir in the eggs. I serve it in a large communal dish with crusty bread. Cilla refuses to eat with her hand, to dip the bread into the soft mixture like I show her. My throat chokes a little on the eggs as I remember the first family lunch, the realisation that Ali and I were to sit at separate tables: the seven men at the large low round table, myself, Ali's mother and little sister Maryam at the smaller one. I didn't have a name for his mother. I tried to call her Khadija, but Ali said not to. I wanted to call her *Muy*, Mum, but I was too shy. I looked across, longing to be near Ali, my interpreter, as their table rang with laughter and jokes and conversation in Arabic. *Muy* occasionally threw what sounded like witty comments across, her round face beaming. At our table, with no common language, we contented ourselves with smiles and glances. Maryam and I waited for *Muy* to begin, then carefully ate from the section of the *tagine* just in front of us. *Muy* moved more vegetables into our territory if our share seemed lacking. She urged us on if we paused in the right-handed movement of bread to plate to mouth. When we had eaten sufficient vegetables, she chose a piece of meat for us, breaking it up with her hand.

After the *chachouka* I change into the white embroidered *fokia* Ali gave me: the kaftan that Moroccan men wear, a perfect nightdress. Once Ali wore it on our after-dinner walk in Cairo, with his *babouches*, grey pointy Moroccan slippers. I put on the *djelliba* he picked for me,

123

the traditional hooded outer-garment. Ali said the silver colour went with my eyes. I have saved it for you, wrapped in brown paper. As we walked through the heaving Friday-night crowds on Sharia al-Ahram, everybody stared, but then everybody always stared at us, Westerner and Arab. 'They are admiring our clothes,' Ali said. 'They are asking, is she French? And conferring, she is French.'

I enjoyed it: the dress-ups, the mistaken identity, so much a part of travelling for me. In India I wore a *shalwar kameez* of bright iridescent green. I pulled my hair back tightly, lined my eyes with kohl and wore a bindi. In Fort Cochin a local man said I looked like a Kashmiri woman, and I was pleased. Often I think travel is just a grown-up game of pretend. Trying on other lives.

I know you are there at your cousin's nativity play. You revealed yourself, a strip of blue, in the white plastic wand I had waved around in disbelief. The tiredness much more than jetlag. Camille is one of the usual surfeit of five-year-old angels. She looks scared on stage and at first her mouth merely opens and closes on the Christmas carols. The scene could be from my own childhood except for more Asian faces. I try to insert you there. Would you feel left out? Would Ali not want you to take part? I am fixated by the veiled Mary, the turbaned Joseph, the wise men, all dressed like the Egyptians and Moroccans so recently left behind. The scene, representing 1999 years before, could easily be now, there. With the Three Kings in Nikes and a satellite TV in the corner, blasting out programmes from around the Arab world.

We talked about having children, strolling along the palm-lined paths of Kho Phi Phi, discussing names. I was enchanted with the fairytale-like Arabic names which Ali explained often conjured up the pleasing aspects of nature at the time of birth. Qamar, Maham and Badriya referred to the moon, Suha, Thuraya and Zahra to the stars, Leila to night. Or they could suggest decent qualities – Ali mentioned two brothers whose names meant loyalty and generosity, his father whose name meant happy. He hoped to call our first son Samir, he said – warm breeze: that would be a fine day, for sure.

They could be brought up as Muslims, if he wanted, I said airily. Ali didn't even pray. He said they could choose. I thought of it as a cultural backdrop, as Catholicism had been for me. Something to question, and perhaps rebel against, subjecting the skies to intense scrutiny, as I had after catechism classes, looking for signs.

It was OK for Ali to marry a Jew or a Christian because we were People of the Book, like Muslims, he explained. But never a Hindu, or a Buddhist. If I was a man and he a woman, I'd have to convert: a non-Muslim man couldn't marry a Muslim woman. 'That's not fair,' I said. 'Lucky for you, my beauty,' he laughed, 'you can have me for your husband,' and dived under the water. We were on a tropical island then, swimming in the warm Andaman Sea. Ali loved the water: he swam until his toes wrinkled. I told him I didn't know what I believed in. 'I believe in trees, I believe in sky,' I shouted into the blue expanse above. Every night we swam from our rock at one end of the village. Then we showered and walked along the paths to dinner, arm-in-arm. I drank a beer and he drank a Coke, and our differences didn't matter, neither of us inside our own culture.

I gaze at the Three Kings gazing adoringly at the Child Jesus. What if you are a boy? Will you have to be taught that men are superior? I'm excited by the idea of a naming ceremony on your seventh day, the colourful, unfamiliar rituals, but what about when you are four? Would you be surprised one day like Ali, a big party in your honour and then the release of white doves? You look up, enchanted, and then there is a sharp pain and you look down and you are bleeding. They bandage you up and ride you around and around on a donkey, high up, and you are so excited you scarcely feel the pain. What if you are damaged? What if we go and live in Morocco and your grandmother consults a *fakir* for a problem with your health? Like when his older brother died and Ali became sickly, and the *fakir* burnt a bald spot into his scalp to get rid of evil influences.

As Camille begins to sing for real, finally looking happy, I don't comprehend how to have a child with a different childhood from mine. I have read that the children of Muslim men are automatically considered Muslim. Christmas or Ramadan, how will you choose? Ali said you could. Why am I so worried? Isn't it simply about our sweetest childhood memories, wanting to pass the feelings on? The wonderment of Ali's doves; the fun of decorating a Christmas tree.

You won't believe I was ever a young woman. When you read this, I will be fifty-one. I imagine I will have let my hair go white by then. 'I want to let my hair go white, like an angel,' I said to my sisters, who hovered about me in shock after I found out about Ali. I imagined lying in the bathtub, my white hair floating out around me, a vision of sorrow, my still-young face and the floating wavy hair. 'My young husband,' I said over and over again, like I was already an old woman. You won't believe how black my hair was once – so black, men would turn me into their fantasy Latin lover: Spanish, Italian, French, not suspecting my Irish roots. You won't believe anyone ever fantasised like that about me, or that my skin was once a fine white, like a mask stretched over my face.

When I met your father it was not so fine; I was already in my thirties, but you won't believe me when I say I still considered myself a young woman. A young woman with a past, but still hopeful. I suppose it sounds either terribly romantic or terribly trashy that I met your father in Bangkok in the last half of the last year of the last century. Who knows what has happened to that noisy, dirty but vehemently living city? Whether yellow *tuk tuks* still roar up and down its congested streets and monks dress in saffron robes, smoking furtive cigarettes and following Manchester United on the BBC World Service. Neither Ali nor I had been living in the place we came from. We were displaced people, trying to find somewhere to belong: pick a guidebook and go. I was waiting for a visa to India. Ali had been trying to get to Iceland.

'I'm a Third World Citizen,' he said bitterly, 'so they would not give me a visa. I can only get visas to Third World countries, like Thailand. You are so lucky, you can go anywhere. First World Citizen.'

You wouldn't have been born if there wasn't a last empty seat at my table. If it wasn't Ali's favourite noodle stall. I barely glanced at him when he asked to sit down. Just another young backpacker. He looked to me like an Israeli: curly dark hair, brown eyes, lightly tanned skin, tall. I had let streaks of premature grey stay in my temples in the hope of being treated like a wise woman in India, not a sexual object to be harassed. In my bag I kept a photo of my brother with Camille and me. 'My husband and daughter,' I would say if anyone asked, so no one would feel sorry for me in that family-obsessed culture. 'I'm meeting them tomorrow,' I'd say.

If I hadn't been so clumsy opening the cheap Thai water bottle, we would never have spoken. Your father's face across the table as he helped me was a boy's face; an impression of sweet rounded cheeks which were somehow no longer there when we finally made full eye-contact. He looked like such a boy, and I have said I considered myself still a young woman. But not a woman who was going to fall in love again, not with a foreigner. And certainly not with a boy. I was travelling once more before finally making my home in Australia, finally settling down, and one day I was sure I would have you in my arms, a baby of my own. I just knew I had to cultivate patience.

I couldn't believe Ali was Moroccan: shouldn't he be small and dark, and speak broken English? He mistook me for an Italian; I was dressed modestly and not full of body piercings, he said approvingly, like all the English girls. And Australian girls were all big and strong, as if they worked on a farm, he insisted. It wasn't love at first sight but we couldn't stop talking.

We fell in love the next night, *bang*, sitting by the Chao Phraya. Your father spoke to me in all his seductive tongues: French, Spanish, Italian, Arabic, Tashelit and his delightful English with its formal French idioms. It was the words, and the hot night, and the brown river, and the surrealness of the jetty where homeless people slept. Instead of finding a riverside restaurant, we stumbled upon this quiet dirty corner. Behind us the expressway roared; two old men lay talking on uncomfortable benches; lit-up junk barges glided by, rocking the wooden jetty; young Thai couples came and went. Each new arrival whispered *farang, farang*, foreigner, to each other. We weren't hungry or thirsty. We sat for hours, swapping stories, equally startled by the other's strange details: my First Communion, dressed like a tiny bride in white dress and veil; his circumcision, magical white doves flung into the air. As we talked I began to imagine a Moroccan wedding, ridiculous, but that's how quickly I fell in love with him. With me held high above the crowd on the wedding chair.

Five weeks later, I flew from London to Malaga, took a bus through Spain, and caught the boat to Tangier. We planned to marry in October. I was coming to meet his family. 'They already love you,' Ali said.

In letters to my family, I tried to explain how I could fall in love so quickly, agree to marry a stranger. I wrote: *Everybody loves him because he is kind and smiling and laughing. The Thai stall-holders adore him. He sits half the day with one young man who sells books; he makes friends easily. To a homesick Moroccan he sang fifty-six Arabic songs in a row to cheer him up; he spent most of the day singing to him. The man said he was the best friend he had ever had. He sings to me, in Tashelit and Arabic, even English and French. He sings to me! He is very generous – if you said you liked something he would give it to you.*

His passions and friendships are fast and fleeting, his love of songs and words enduring. I am sorry he never sung a song to you, *habibetet.*

'It is too soon,' he says, calling to tell me this on Christmas Day. 'People will think we had to get married.' This was unacceptable to Muslims. This carried shame, *hshuma*, threatening the honour of his family. 'I want my family to respect our marriage. I am not a baby machine. I am not a sex machine.'

I'm shocked at his coldness, but feel excruciatingly sympathetic. So sorry for him. Our love offered him the chance to be a First World Citizen, which was his dream, to freely travel anywhere, do anything. We could live in England, I said, we could live in France. We would go to Iceland, he would finally see the land of ice, of snow and all-day summer. I still wanted these things for him.

Once Ali said, if he was wronged, he cut people dead, just like that. He never spoke to them again. Did a wife fall into this category?

\* \* \*

129

Too panicked to face what is happening, I take the phone off the hook.

I spend New Year's Eve with my family on the harbour, shivering on a sandstone ledge overlooking Rose Bay, the national park behind us. Raining and cold, the weather mirroring the mood of a tragedy, not the summer Sydney I remember. Wanting to reread *Macbeth* before midnight, I separate myself on a further rock, pleading nausea. I've told them about you already, as if to protect you from harm, from a decision a Catholic family won't respect. Two can play at his game. They drink champagne, I drink ginger beer. I copy out 'Time and the hour run through the roughest day'. I look at Ali's photo at midnight, but it's not the same. A huge gap seems to have opened up between us, wider than the span of the Harbour Bridge, which looks as if it's exploding. Burst after burst of fireworks, enough noise to scream my heart out and not be heard, silhouettes of huge startled birds, pelicans and ibis, flung up in terror from the bush and the bay. Then the calm lingering word in burning copperplate: *Eternity*.

When I get home, I put the phone back on the receiver.

On the first day of the twenty-first century, a call comes, from 1420, from another culture, another world. It tells me that I am divorced, dispensed with, handed back to my own family. Ali doesn't repeat it three times, like the stories you hear. I'm not a Muslim, not even a believer – it matters very much now that I believe in trees, in sky. 'What would we teach our children?' he asks. I am *harram*, taboo, like unclean food. 'It was all a mistake, I was weak.' He has already married his cousin. He is going to Kuwait to work, taking her with him. He wants a good Muslim wife.

'But you're married to me,' I say. He has married his own *cousin*? I don't understand, he's my husband, we spent two months in Cairo trying to get married. I repeated words I didn't understand in the registry office, but we made up our vows when we came home and exchanged our rings.

I hang up. I wonder how many times he has slept with his virgin cousin, whether she too is already pregnant. My morning nausea rises. I think, in-breeding. I imagine half-brothers and sisters with twisted genes, one eye lower, stick-out ears, a hare-lip, a club foot. I remember his brother Jamahl's remark: 'Girls are tender chickens, waiting to be plucked.' I feel rescued. I feel devastated. I feel angry. But most of all I feel sorry for you. I cry for two days and then I begin to bleed. I stop crying, I remain calm, and you cling on.

Your daddy won't reply now, won't acknowledge you. His brothers, who were so kind, who wished peace be with me, hands on their hearts, scorn me when I ring up. Poor little half-Moroccan baby who won't have a daddy, who won't have a brother or a sister who looks like you. No naming ceremony after seven days, everyone coming and sleeping on the floor and feasting in your honour. Not five funny uncles and two pretty aunts with long dark wavy hair. We don't know any Arab people. We don't know any Arab songs. I've forgotten what these words mean, that your father taught me to sing in the Andaman Sea: *fuli mae fookai a habibi habibi*. Only *habibi* – beloved. I make *couscous* from a packet but it comes out lumpy. My mint tea is OK, though, sweet, green and refreshing. Not as strong as your grandfather's: the mint-tea ritual before dinner, *baba* reclining on cushions, dressed in his comfortable *fokia*, tending the small portable stove, bunches of moist green mint beside him. He pours the first glass of his potent brew in a theatrical arch from the silver teapot on legs, tastes it, pours it back into the pot, waits, then pours in loops into the waiting glasses.

Memories assault me, stabs before I go to sleep, punches as I walk to buy milk. Under the shower, I worry about the radio programme on the dangerous level of pesticides on vegetables in Egypt. In the steamy bathroom, my hair wet, body stinging from a bumpy swim in the surf, I pick the final pieces of sand from my swollen nipples, rub oil on my growing belly. We ate loads of vegetables in Cairo, they seemed so vigorous and healthy, piled up high in the greengrocer's, opposite the place where we bought our chickens. Customers arranged for them to be killed. I remember the first one, still warm when Ali brought it upstairs. And very tender. Sometimes they had goats tethered outside, bleating, and then you would see blood on the street later, and the goat hanging upside down.

You cling on, but I try not to get too attached. I can't feel you yet, you are only sickness and tiredness, sorrow. At fourteen weeks I have a scan, and there you are, a huge head, two arms and legs and even little hands. You make these flick-flip movements like a giant hiccup. My parasite, hidden cargo from Cairo. Seeing you, a feeling of being thawed out, allowed to love you. Allowed to feel some hope. Afterwards, at the beach, I unpeel a banana and eat it slowly, a gift for you, deep in your unconscious growing. I stare at the young bodies lying on the sand, awed at the beginnings of such a body within me.

I sleep well and deeply for the first time in weeks. Then I am awakened after giving birth, you tightly swaddled beside me. There is no memory of the birth, no pain. I lean over you, only a tiny section of your face visible; even your brow wrapped, like a tiny Muslim woman, scarved. Your dark brows are knit in the anxious expression I have seen on your grandmother when she is making Friday's *couscous*, concentrating, caught unawares. You have the same round chubby cheeks. I am a little frightened of your half-submerged face, so fierce, the expression, so Moroccan: little old peasant woman, are you angry at me? Will you love me? I begin to unwrap the bundle. I start with your head and when I remove your veil, you fix me with such dark, long-lashed eyes. You are smiling Ali's wide smile and it doesn't stab me, it fills me with a strange forgotten feeling: happiness. I continue unwinding and examine you slowly, count your fingers, see your swollen vulva, and cry with joy that you are a girl. Then a nurse comes in and says there is a problem with your foot, and I say, 'Yes, her Uncle Aziz had a club foot,' but I don't feel worried. She massages your foot and it is fine. Then you are naked and I just hold you.

My real awakening finds my arms crossed over my chest and a feeling of calm through my whole body.

I am no longer afraid of you: what sharp memories you might bring me. Unwrapped, totally naked, outside any culture, you will be waiting to be imprinted with your own memories, you will arrive brand new.

One day I look at my grey hair in the mirror, the streaks making me grave before my time, and I dye my hair dark again. I begin to recover. When it is autumn, I see pomegranates on sale in the corner shop. *Rammen*, they're called in Morocco. I am amazed to see them here, the tough pinky skin, rising to the spiky tuft where Ali would bite the fruit open with his teeth. I didn't like the bitter taste of the skin, the squirt of pink staining juice that his skilled method avoided. 'Look, you can see her eyes,' he always said when he first revealed the pink gems within. 'She is a beauty, this one.'

'Eating *rammen*, it's one of our hobbies,' I joked once in Cairo, as we sat after dinner intently peeling and eating the fruit, seed by seed.

I am brave enough to buy one. I don't faint or reel when I hold its familiar weight and roundness in my hand.

Your inheritance shall be a taste for pomegranate, your father's favourite fruit. We will call them *rammen* between ourselves. If you also have his smile, and love to sing me songs, I will be blessed. 'Look, you can see her eyes,' I tell you as the pink juice spurts and stains the sand with my clumsy opening technique. I will never be as good at it as your father. I sit in my costume, my legs in yoga cobbler pose, soles of my feet flat against each other, training my pelvis to open up, to bear you. I carefully peel and separate the segments, eat each tiny jewel one by one.

# The Whole of Europe

## *Bridget O'Connor*

Ruth held the phone away from her ear but the voice was still spiralling down the dog-chewed telephone wire. 'What?' she said. 'What did you say?' The bad news had made her temporarily deaf. Mary, friend of her youth, was having twins.

'Twins,' Ruth mouthed, feeling a double body blow, first – *pow!* – on her temple then straight – *wham*! – in her guts. Twins. Two. That was more than one. Double. Greedy. 'Wow.' Her voice went up a tone. 'That's *fan* . . . wow! Is Dan pleased?' 'Yes, Dan is,' Mary said. Then, she was shouting: 'Ruth, he's OVER THE MOON. He's gone straight out to buy TWO giant teddy bears and TWO of those mega-Yorkie bars. And . . .' Her voice went on. Something about the spare room and wanting to move and that old moany bitch downstairs and, more faintly, 'It will be your turn next.' Ruth felt bile rise in her stomach. A tide of something else washed over her too, so strong she had to lean her forehead on the foggy window-pane. It's happy people, she thought, they make me sick. 'Ah, that's great news,' she managed and cooed down the phone.

*Coo coo lucky you.*

She had a headache for the rest of the day. 'It's migraine,' she told work. She said out loud, 'Fuck the payroll.' And spent the day at the Odeon crying through *You've Got Mail*. She was thirty-eight.

'Thirty-eight ain't so old,' her Assistant Payroll Manager/works-best-friend Annie said loudly, in the cardboard skyscraper, the next day. 'Not if you want to M&C.' She stood up to yell across the office, modelling, on the way, her new snakeskin pink plastic skirt. 'Oi, Sally. Is thirty-eight too old to Meet & Conceive? Nah, that's what I said . . .' Ruth had to shush her down. 'What?' Annie said. Then, with a roll of her popped blue eyes, 'What *now*? I'm only saying you're not young-young – true – but thirty-eight is like the new twenty-eight. Am I right, Sal? Am I?' No, you're *wrong*, Ruth thought, and snapped a pencil in half. Annie was just twenty-two. Nothing was too old for her. Or too young. They had to face each other all day. I've shared too much, Ruth thought. I've leaked.

But she couldn't help herself.

The day was too long.

And there it was again, lurching across her belly, a tide of something, like sea-sickness.

*Twins*.


'It's all geography anyway,' Annie said, after fag-break, the next day. 'E numbers. N numbers.' She went on. She could type and talk. She paused to study her new leopard-skin acrylic fingernails. Three inches. 'Nice, in't they?' Ruth lived in E5. No good. 'You should move to N16.' Tap tap tap. 'Ain't that right, Sal? N16 has the highest ratio of Under Fives in the whole of Europe. It rains sperm there,' she said. She was completely deadpan. 'I'm serious. It happens in clusters, you know, like in those childhood leukaemia cases? Did you see that old film about the spooky blonde kids in the village – you know, widows and virgins had them. Old maids were taken . . . well, they were ever so surprised.'

Annie was loyal, Ruth reminded herself on the way home. Persistent anyway, the way she just *kept on* plugging away at Ruth's favourite subject; lined up potential

M&Cs she – somehow – located throughout the crêpy fluorescent layers of the cardboard skyscraper. She spent their lunch-hour reading from the Lonely Hearts column, de-coding: 'WANTED: TLK FOR MDA – what do you think that means? Talkative? Lesbian? Kind? CONVICTED FELON SEEKS LADYFRIEND. MUST HAVE GSOH – wotcha think?' But Ruth sometimes had to turn her sound down. She pulled her collar up and pressed on through her malodorous treeless neighbourhood, passing the launderette/youth club, the Knackered Kurdish Bread shop, the pub with the fifty-year-old strippers, the black hole where the cashpoint machine once was, the barren lands of E5. Maybe I *should* move, Ruth thought, but the thought didn't last too long.

'Babies/labies,' her mother said on the phone after Ruth had told her about Mary. 'Twins, hey.' Her mother had a fag-pause while she wound herself up. 'Well, girl, you've missed that boat. You had your chance. Am I right? I'm right, aren't I? Am I right? Am I? Say it?' 'Yes, Mum,' Ruth nodded. 'You're right.' She was. Her mother's voice went up a whine. 'I mean, Ruth, didn't *you* and Dan once have some kind of . . . thing?'

They had.

Twins.

It could have been her. She felt the snap of Polaroids. The whirr of the ciné-camera. She saw Dan waving at her in blurry Technicolor.

*Dan and Ruth.*

*Dan and Ruth pictured here with wee Danny and Ruthie.*

*In the people-carrier.*

*The double buggy.*

*Seen here at the park. The beach. Tucked up in their bunk-beds.*

*And pictured here too with fond family friend Auntie Mary.*

She spent the evening drinking vodka in the utility/nursery room, ironing a stack of work blouses, pressing the sleeves flat, steaming the smile from fat Mary's fecund robbing face.

And woke with her ears full of tears. This must stop, Ruth told herself in the shower. She was becoming one of those women. The ones Annie took the piss out of via email. Hormonal, permanently pre-menstrual, easily, so easily undone. Like Miss Dorset in Personnel. She cried if she dropped a ruler. Or the Cat Woman Tina O'Leary in Dockets and Damages: she had framed cat photos on her desk – plus a number, it was rumoured (by Annie), of furry unnatural relationships. Or Gail Lansman, the Under-the-Secretary, who had been seen crying alone in her Peugeot in the company car park. 'Shuddering,' Annie had said, 'tarty sobs.'

Ruth put on her Manager's face; it was orange, slightly streaky, and opened the door. Outside the day wobbled. She set her chin firmly. But it was already too late.

At work she lifted Annie's in-tray closer, barked a series of managerial, slightly crazed, hung-over commands and watched her own reflection form on her olive-green computer screen, till that was all she saw. Behind the scroll of figures she was wispy, transparent. When she frowned suddenly, her face fell in. I should have married Alan, she thought, lifting her hands off the keyboard for a moment, pushing them through her sticky managerial bob, my university sweetheart. I should have stopped myself right there. Just, as my mother said:

Stopped.

Yourself. Young lady.

And kept.

Still.

Oh don't, Ruth counselled herself, go there, girl. But too late. She'd already gone.

Alan had been bearded, bookish, sexually extreme. Or that's what she'd thought at the time. He was like a line drawing in a sex manual. Methodical. Mechanical. Obscene. She should have stuck with him or *any* one of the men she'd stacked up in her twenties – Keiran, Sean, Des, Dan – men who would when she would not. They were all married now, fat or just plain fucked. Or they'd bred out like, Ruth shuddered deeply, Joe: that same faint chin shrinking to nothing on his row of kids. Or Anthony, starring now in *Repeat of the Monobrow*. Or in Keiran's case, Ruth suddenly felt weepy, though she'd never actually liked him all that much, they had died.

'Fag?' Annie said, waving her Marlboro full tar in front of Ruth's face. She was still young enough for full strength. Ruth shook her head and typed faster. She typed away. Through Elevenses. Twelvesies. Into blur. She typed THIRTY-EIGHT IS OLD. Then a row of question-marks. But, indisputably – and who would argue – her eggs *were* old.

Test.

Would she buy her own eggs in a supermarket?

She sent a virtual self tapping off down an aisle.

No.

She went tapping right past Old Eggs to Farm Fresh. Then she was checking out the Free Range, reading the tiny pink tattoo date with a buyer's slow-to-satisfy beaming smile. Her eggs were old. Each month she could hear their suicide notes, a kind of granular groan, as they plopped to their death down her uterus. AHHHHHH. Then AHH-THANK-THE-FUCK. She was crispy-eyed too, especially after a laugh. Ruth tried a laugh. HA HA HA HA. Then she tried it out loud. It rang over the hum of the air conditioning, made Sally, who was pert and thirty, whiz round twice on her spinning chair. Then she stopped it dead.

And stared.

She was right. Her screen image was *still* wrinkled a full minute later. She leaned closer till all she saw was eye-wet. And . . . cracks. Each birthday brought a new detail like that. She had squeaky bones, a new fold at the neck. Hands that were, she looked at hers clawing away at the keyboard, speckled and veined like two sparrow eggs.

She should have married Keiran. She'd be a widow by now with 2.4 kids. She'd be going to a gym toning up for sex not procreation, thinking about vehicles and vaccinations, Range Rovers and mumps. But who knew? Who knew she would end up alone and – Ruth closed her eyes tight – *feeling like this?*

'I found this bloke for you,' Annie said at lunchtime in the park the next day. She took her headphones off and plumped up her electrocuted pink fringe. A sparrow flew by, looping the loop in the smudgy grey and peach sky. Ruth watched it veer suddenly into a tree of cobwebby nests, saw brown beaks gawp up, heard a tiny orchestra of squeaks. Twins. Doubled. No, it was quads. A cold feeling ran down her neck.

'What's wrong with him,' she said, 'this bloke?' She took a prawn out of her sandwich, sniffed it, then threw it at a duck.

Missed.

'Nothing,' Annie said. 'Well,' she lit a fag, 'nothing visible anyway. Hold on a sec. Two o'clock. Ugly Baby Alert! Ah my . . . it's ginger . . . *gross*!'

His name was Rolf. Rolf Mitchel. Head of Marketing and Development. He was coming soon, fresh from the Harrow and Wealdstone branch. Annie's email spy had described him as 'cute with a clipboard. You know, the rolled-up-sleeve kind?' Ruth did know. Sometimes she thought, I know too much.

\*     \*     \*

'It is *not* a dog's name,' Annie snapped.

They were spying on Rolf Mitchel, two days later, through the tinted glass of the training wing. Annie looked peeved suddenly; her lip ledged out, the way it did when the computers crashed and she'd run out of strawberry lip-gloss. I must be trying, Ruth thought. I must be a right pain in the . . . but she couldn't stop. She was going on, on and on, boring the same black-hole. And it was only two o'clock, grey and rainy outside. She could feel the sway of the weather under the cardboard floor. The long second-ticking day. She said, in a more conciliatory tone, 'And how old is he, anyway?' but Annie didn't know.

She doesn't *have* to know, Ruth thought, and watched the man at the front of the class point at a flipchart full of squares and arrows. The people around him nodded and made notes. He looked thirty-five but Ruth wasn't fooled. The glass they were spying through was tinted the same age-defying bronze found in aeroplane loos and certain hair-dressing salons. You wouldn't mind dying if you looked like that. You wouldn't mind being cut up by trainees. 'More,' you'd cry, 'shorter, shorter,' till you were revealed in broad daylight, bald and wrinkled, old. He could be forty-five – fifty? He was probably panting into late middle-age, dragging his knackered seed bag behind him. 'Rolf,' Ruth said, under her breath. Then she rolled her R's, but very quietly so tetchy Annie wouldn't hear: '*Rolf-Rolf. Rolf Rolf.*' The man looked up. He cocked his head. He really *was*, Ruth decided, dog-like. He had shaggy black hair. His legs were too short for his body. He gave a corporate laugh suddenly so loud they could hear it through the glass. 'He's got a lot of teeth,' Ruth said, peering in further under her hand. 'Teeth is good,' Annie said. She wheeled round. She gave Ruth her injured pop-eyed look. 'You said the last one had too much hair.'

'Indisputably,' Ruth said.

Because it was true. Mike, 'call me Mickey', Floor 13, Assistant Head of Personnel and Head of Paper Clip Chains, he did have funny hair. As she'd explained to Annie, at length, day after day, you couldn't give a kid a father like that. As a would-be parent you had Responsibilities. It would be practically a war crime. He had hair like a load of knuckles, Ruth had said, in a row. Rows and rows of tiny clenching fists. At the cinema she'd heard the bones settling and clicking all around his head. The one before that, Henry, Floor 2, something to do with Import Law and pink felt-tip pens, he'd had a widow's hump and a sinister silent laugh. They'd had one long drink after work. How would she know if he was being humorous, she'd said to Annie afterwards? He wasn't any good at telling jokes. Men in their late thirties/early forties – they told stories now, long long long long stories, not jokes. You had to search their faces for a punch-line. *If* there was one. Because, very often, they were only telling you about something that *moved* them. Like from their childhood. And they were always finding things 'moving'. Who knew? She'd hear his shoulders shaking on the pillow. He could be crying or having a heart attack and she'd feel compelled to join in and laugh just in case. What if it was an inherited condition? What kind of mother would that make her? The one before that, Tim, one of the execs on the top floor, he'd had a long soft nose like a parsnip and too much body hair. He must have shaved his hands and wrists, his nose, for work but she'd seen a slit of black rug through his Paul Smith date shirt. The one before that . . . 'Tick tock,' Annie said. 'Get our Miss Choosy,' and she looked at Ruth, suddenly showing her youth.

Ruth thought, I could have you fired.

And heard the seconds collide in the carpet-stinky air.

'Forgetaboutit,' she said instead, and they went down in separate lifts and launched the payroll, watching the scroll of green numbers flash and kick out digital light against their cheeks.

'G'night, then,' Annie mumbled when the clock had, eventually, lurched its way down to home-time, pulling on her long scarlet fake-fur coat. 'Night,' Ruth said, and busied herself, cheeks burning, in her top drawer till Annie's heels, followed by pert Sally's heels, followed by the rest of the office drones, had clicked and clacked away. I am alone, Ruth thought, and felt the lights go out, snapping off right through her, floor by crêpy floor.

On the bus home she found Rolf's phone number in her purse. Annie must have smuggled it there. She saw it as she flashed her pass and squeezed herself in between two podgy sets of pinstriped thighs. Annie must have smuggled it there when I went to the loo, Ruth thought, eyes smarting at the thought of the long afternoon she'd just endured, humped behind her computer, imagining the acid emails Annie was launching under her animal nails. By now she'd be one of those women. Rubbished in cyber-space. She'd be up there with Tina O'Leary, the Cat Woman who 'loves pussy', sobbing beside Gail Lansman in her Peugeot, carted off like Miss Dorset to the rest room whenever her extension line rang. Stop it, Ruth told herself. But she saw the email go bold – '**Warning. Old Ruth wants a baby**' – then spring into upper case. 'RUTH= BARREN. IS DESPERATE. IS SPERM MAGNET. JUST CALL PAY-ROLL. EXT: 230 . . .'

Annie had written ROLF on a yellow Post-it note, then the digits, then a shaky pink felt-tipped heart stuffed with an arrow. It's a peace offering, Ruth thought, or is it, her eyes narrowed, a declaration of war? But she couldn't afford to think like that. The day was too long. And Annie was probably just being, well, Annie: persistent. Above all, young. And this Rolf, he might well be a really nice bloke. He might well be, Ruth blinked, the future father of my child. 'Rolf,' she murmured. She held his name in her mouth for a while, rolled it, humming, over three sleeping policemen, six bus stops. Rolf. ROLFFFFFFFFFFFFFFFFFFFFFFFFF.

ROLF.

But it felt . . . wrong.

She tried again.

Ruth and Rolf. Rolf and Ruth. Little Rolfy. *Hey Ruth, what are you and Rolf doing on Saturday?* A man with a dog's name. Rolf Mitchel. Mitch? Mitchy. *Mitch! Here, boy.* She heard Rolf panting in the corner of a room. Then he was showing the length of his black and scarlet gums, grizzling his side-teeth, looking at her with his mournful dog eyes, pointing a paw at a clipboard. She might give birth to a puppy. She might drop a whole litter of . . . snouts. Ruth clicked her purse shut and pushed out suddenly into the rain.

And found she'd got off the bus way too early. For a long head-turning moment she was lost in space. It was just as though a soft hood of darkness had fallen briefly over her face. She pulled it off. Where was the Sucked-Out Fruit Shop? The Dead Man's Pawn Shop? The Crime Scene Kebab shops of E5? Her heart skipped a beat. *Texture* read one sign. *Interiors* said another. *Babyland* said a third. She was surrounded by purple cafés done out like caves, designer toy shops, a shop that featured just the one spot-lit Baby gro. She was in the village of . . . Stoke Newington. N16. She was standing bareheaded in the baby-making rain. Ruth snorted. Then she laughed the rest of her short crisp laugh. HA HA HA! In the whole of Europe. Here she was, dropped down. In the whole of spooky fucking Europe. . . . She'd tell Annie in the morning, break the ice. She'd . . . Then she heard it. A smothered sound. Something deep and wide was coming at her. Rolling hard through the dark rain. And there they were.

Old mothers in macs, a wrinkled army, marching three abreast, taking the pavement with their chins, pushing their prams and their go-cart-shaped pushchairs, their babies and toddlers a pink and grey scrawl, pawing up through the murk of their plastic rain shields. It will pass, Ruth thought, as she found herself buffeted into the gutter. One day. One day I won't want this any more.

It was time to stop. Young Lady.

Stop. And.

Just. Be.

Still.

Ruth stood very still for a moment in the gluey rain.

Then she pulled up her collar and made her way home.

'You have just the one new message,' her answer-machine service sneered.

Ruth stood dripping at the centre of her empty flat. She had just the one message from Mother. Not so much a message, she thought, wiping her hair on a tea-towel, as a high-pitched whining noise. Rolf could probably hear that. Then she checked her email, one eye on the TV page, the vodka bottle standing alone in its own arctic-blue light, an ear cocked to the grainy silence in her flat. Perhaps she should get a cat this time. (Her last pet, a toy poodle, had jumped from the window and died.) 'You have just the one new message,' her email service said. It was a message from Mary and Dan, friends of her youth. They'd sent a duplicate message to 'all our friends'. I'll read it tomorrow, Ruth thought, but found her eyes were already decoding the screen. Mary had written (it would be Mary, Dan didn't do, Ruth remembered, exclamations), 'OH LOOK!!!! LOOK AT OUR LOVELY LITTLE BABIES!!!!!!!!!!!'

Ruth looked.

She saw a scanned-in picture of Mary's scan. Two ghostly figures in a grey oceanic swirl. She heard the pound and slosh of the ultrasound. Then they were flooding the screen, rising through her belly.

*Twins*.

One moment later Ruth was on the carpet, grabbing at her purse and the yellow Post-it note.

'Rolf?' she said. 'Rolf? Is that you, Rolf?

'Will you put Rolf on the phone, please? I'd like to speak to Rolf. Is that you, Rolf? Rolf? Rolf? Rolf? Rolf?'

She was practically barking into the phone.

# Table of Events

## *Christopher Cyrill*

### 1997

The mousetrap wakes me. X has her back to me but I feel that she too is awake. Her stomach heaves like a moored ship. The mouse will be dead or dying. I don't want to know.

For 2 weeks I had heard it scratching behind the boards of the fireplace, had heard the spillage in the cupboard. It gnawed through the rubber band on the sultanas, ate through the cardboard box containing the breadsticks. 2 nights I baited the trap with sultanas and cream cheese. Last night I baited and set.

In a moment – I know what X will say, in a moment – she will say, 'It's a bad sign.'

I prepare my arguments – its shit could poison the child, food costs money, it's only a fucking mouse. She says nothing and in the morning the mouse, the trap are gone.

Remembered mice:

a) the mouse my father suffocated in a plastic bag

b) Virginia's benign breast tumour which she called a 'mouse'

### 1994

On our first meeting X explains that quarks are thought to be comprised of protons which, along with neutrons, make up the nucleus of an atom. She advises me against imagining quarks as constituents of an atom, the way children are part of a family. Quarks at this stage exist only in a theoretical, almost dream state, and unlike a family cannot be reduced to individual components.

## 1997

X and I await confirmation by ultrasound of the death of the child. On the cover of the *Lancet*, the translucent embryo is fixed in the amniotic fluid. Its eyes meet the gaze of the camera. The photograph is propaganda, I tell myself. It is meant to dissuade abortion. The photographer has stationed the child within the cosmos of the womb. It is without doubt – without doubt it is a divinity – a living organism.

On the ultrasound screen the child looks like a coin in a drain, like a partially unearthed bone. Its heartbeat sounds like Morse code.

## 1976

My father has a saying: '2 means 3.'

If 2 plates break, a 3rd will soon fall. If 2 guests arrive, set 3 plates. 3 unexpected guests on 1 night foretell death. 1 random act or event is accident, remains random. 2 has meaning, pattern, propulsion.

Nothing in recent or ancient family history – the cat dying years after the 2 dogs, his 2 lotto wins 1 October, could dissuade my father or myself from the theory of 3.

## 1997

The doctor in the emergency room is named Carolina. She has a pierced nose and plaited dreadlocks that reach down to her thighs. I think I know her from somewhere – a party, mutual friends. She examines X's blood-spotted underwear. I massage X's feet. Carolina tells us of the statistics of miscarriages (1 in 5) and of the danger time (0–12 weeks). She recommends that X make an appointment for a curettage. She arranges for an ultrasound.

The taxi driver drives us home through wet, unfamiliar streets. The rain has stopped but the gutters still run with water and tree branches criss-cross the pavements. Leaves whip on to the windscreen. X says the pain makes her want to scratch her bones.

'I'm sorry for your troubles,' the cabbie says, as I pay him.

The house seems to smell of blood. I open all the windows as X lies on the bed. She whispers something about the storm being late. I leave her as the wind blows the curtains over the bed and slams doors. I drink whisky, first from the bottle, then from a glass. I drink until I am drunk enough to place myself at the bottom of her bed. I massage her feet. I convince myself that we will try for another baby.

Phrases remembered from that night:
  a) In all likelihood
  b) Death is common


## 1996

One of X's work skills is the ability to organise and deploy in a cost-and-time-efficient manner the movement of ammunition from port to port in a time of war or peace, and in a time of war, the movement of troops. She says she will quit the naval service if a war did begin, though she acknowledges that she is 'marking the gravesites' now.

## 1999

In the Archbald Fountain, water runs down the stone creases of the Minotaur's neck. A tourist poses in front of Diana's bow.

## 1996

X and I live above a Samoan family of 9. The 2nd youngest child is named Marigold. She has no legs. She is mute. She moves around the backyard of the apartment block on a skateboard. Her hands are twisted inward and she pulls herself forward on padded wrists. Some days I go out on to our balcony to smoke and see her wedged against the back fence.

## 1997

X does not want to show me her underwear. I tell her I need to see. I turn them inside out. I see the Pleiades in the pattern of her blood-spots.

## 1995

I wake from a dream of my grandfather. The previous day X and I had applied for a flat in Petersham. We had been living with my father for 4 months. We slept in his bed and he slept on the sofa. I could not have sex if he was in the house. I flat-hunted while X worked. I was on the dole. All our applications so far had been unsuccessful.

The flat was small but a Samoan husband and wife and a few kids lived downstairs in a flat of the same dimensions so I imagined it would be spacious enough for the 2 of us. Further, I joked to X, Tresillian, the mothercraft hospital, was 3 doors down, in case we ever decided to have a baby.

In the dream of my grandfather – I can recall no other dreams of him – I enter an orange house on the edge of grasslands. The house becomes a church amidst grasslands. As I near the vestibule I see my grandfather's face emerge from the colour red. I feel calm. His face is round and without lines of age or worry. His teeth are perfect, though he died toothless. My grandfather tells me that we will get the flat. His hands emerge, held *abahya*. His face becomes that of a strange child.


*1997*

Arguments against having the child:
  a) money
  b) overpopulation
  c) the dream of travel
  d) me


*1995*

I meet X for the 2nd time at the National Gallery in Melbourne. I am down from Sydney to visit my mother's grave. X is attending a seminar on fuzzy logic. I have her aunt's number.

I drop 5 cent pieces into the rectangular pond in front of the gallery. The decayed human face of a stone nymph shimmers above mine in the water. X pulls on my coat. I put out my hand and she shakes it. I say that I want her to see the eternal flame of the War Memorial and as we walk along the sand paths – criss-crossed with palm leaves – I tell her the story of the abandoned child left at the foot of the statue of Weary Dunlop and notice how the autumn light changes the colour of her hair from red to brown to red again. I tell her this. She says it's probably the chemicals in the dye. I touch her hair. I tell her the child was found by a council worker, who later adopted it. The mother was never found, never came forward. I point out the statue to her as we near it. It is orange in the same light. She asks if my story is true or a game. I smile and produce page 1031 of Webster's, the word 'quark' highlighted. She says that other men bring flowers.

Other interesting words page 1031:

a)  Quantico
b)  Qualia
c)  Quanta

## 1997

We fight over the amount of money I spend on alcohol and the state of the bathtub. We fight because we could not afford an ambulance to RPA's emergency ward. We have unspoken fights about the dishes. My unspoken arguments are that I only gave our relationship the length of the lease – 6 months – and that I still loved Virginia.

## 1997

A slamming door wakes us, a vase breaks in the middle of the night.

## 2000

Men are sunbaking on the grass and parishioners are leaving the church across the road. Couples, families, are seated around the Archibald Fountain. Other couples, other families – 1 drunk – are sitting or lying on the park benches that encircle the path that encircles the fountain. The child is running ahead of me.

*1997*

I wonder about the man in the hallway as X moves – with the help of her mother – from shower to birth stool to shower. He has a video camera in his left hand and wears a holster holding a 5- by 6-inch battery from his belt. He leaves blood prints on the carpet.

*1997*

My toes feel stuck together. X has her head out of the window. Her hair sticks to her neck with sweat.

'My wife is pregnant – can you please turn on the air?'

'Window is open,' the cab driver says. I can't place his accent.

'Please, she's sick.'

'Air condition costs moneys, not my cab.'

'I won't pay.'

'I stop.'

X puts her hand on mine and tries to unclench my fist. Her fingers, my fingers, are mottled with blood.

'I'll make it,' she says.

The cab pulls over outside RPA. I get out. I make a note of the driver's licence plates. X rips a 20-dollar bill in half and throws it at him.

*2000*

| | |
|---|---|
| *Playschool* presenters currently in love with: | 2 |
| Overtime hours: | 6 |
| Steiner school: | 68 per fortnight |
| Medicare: | 42+42+42 |
| Unreturned calls: | 8 |

## 1996

Even though we have never mentioned starting a family X tells me she has a nest egg and a glory box. Her mother has saved her 1st booties, and the Big Bird candle – his head is ½ melted – from her 3rd birthday.

## 1997

This too is a dream. The child rarely sleeps. I take her out of bed one night so that X can rest, so that her cracked nipples can heal in her sleep. The child and I look at photographs together. In one photo she is lying on her back. The child in the photograph begins to laugh, holds her hands *abahya*. I see my grandfather's face, then I see Buddha. The face of the dream photograph is Buddha, my grandfather, a child not yet conceived.

## 2000

The child runs toward the Minotaur – Minotaur forever awaiting death – in the Archibald Fountain. She has 20 cents in her hand. She runs ahead but stops every few paces to check that the coin has not fallen, that I am still within her sight.

## 1997

My father looks at me with what I interpret as sorrow when I tell him that X is pregnant, that we are keeping the child. He then shakes my hand and offers to buy me a video camera.

*1997*

X takes my penis in her hand and rubs it against her navel.

*1979*

I trace the evolution of a foetus from a torn encyclopaedia.

*1997*

My mouth opens and moves towards her mouth.

*1979*

Within the Caucasian woman's body I trace the various assertions of limbs, the bubbling of skull.

*1997*

I stretch my neck over her stomach to find her tongue.

*1979*

In week 13, within my tracings, my stiff, nervous hands mangle the developing features of the foetus – the eyes smudge into one, the spine becomes too thick.

*1997*

X feels heavy but I can't resist seeing her on top.

*1979*

In week 13, something goes bad for that baby.

*1997*

I put my fingers in her mouth. X guides my fingers to her nipples.

*2000*

The child presses her face against the TV screen at the moment when X appears at the hospital exit. When she sees herself being placed into the baby capsule she claps. X says she seems intrigued but comfortable with her own doubling, as if to exist simultaneously on video and in the living room were simply part of the world not yet defined, as mysterious as fridge magnets, the jack-in-the-box.

*1997*

X's list of bad signs:
   a) lack of morning sickness
   b) stomach cramps 3-hourly
   c) liver pains
   d) craving cream cheese

*1997*

In the ultrasound photo the child is in profile. I have left my fingerprint upon one dark corner. I tell X that the child looks like my grandfather. She laughs.

*1997*

Personal list of bad signs:
   a) the occurrence of the word 'letheward' in a text
   b) blackouts

c) crow sightings in multiples of 3
d) carcasses on bitumen

## 2000

The baby zig-zags towards the child and me. X is close by her. The child has made her wish but, knowing the mysterious, fragile logic of wishing, is keeping the secret. Pedestrians are dodging the baby as she investigates leaves, discarded champagne corks. They are approaching us haphazardly, along the arcade made by the meeting of fig-tree branches, in a dappled light.

## 1997

My hands shake and I do not like to drive. My father is bringing the baby home. I vacuum and dust. I replace old bulbs with bulbs of lesser wattage. I place locks on the cutlery drawer, move the household poisons – washing powder, whisky – beyond even the reach of X. I knot plastic bags, knot curtain cords. The child's cot is as bare as a fallen nest. The flat is quiet except for a scratching in the floorboards.

# Gwendolyn

## *Alice Jerome*

Gwendolyn Pound did not stir from the lair of her futon.

A bowl of cornflakes had been placed on the floor and Gwendolyn's hand was hanging an inch above it, swaying gently with her breathing. Meanwhile Wesley had to go. Wes had known he was going for a week, but knew these things are like little deaths and now he must get on. His face, usually so round and kind, assembled itself into a face that disguised disappearance.

He watched her milky lids open slowly, her dark blue eyes looking at him from the absorption of a thick dream. Her slender hand covered her face, and her long legs stretched and swam under the thin sheet, as if she was aware of him already. Then she sat up quickly, the long blonde hair falling. He remembered one dark raining afternoon, when he still hardly knew her but wanted to be inside her all the time, she had said, 'Hair down to your waist at thirty-five can only be a secret inside out.' He understood she was expecting him to understand, so he hadn't asked.

Wes wasn't interested any more, he reminded himself as he zipped his jacket. But he did remember when he leaned on her hair with his elbows and she would give a small smiling cry, and when it covered him.

Gwen stood up, and he felt her presence almost sadly, knowing he was leaving.

'I thought it was time you got up – it's twelve. I'm sort of going, going to Paris about a job that Monique knows

*158*

about. I'm meeting this journalist she says is fearless and we could be going to Alaska. In two weeks if it works out. I'm sorry, I know it's short notice, I only knew this morning.'

'I see. And when can I expect you back? At all?' She pulled her nightie over her head.

Wes ruminated around his body for some sexual desire. There was the erotic charge of knowing something she did not, but he couldn't bear the required warmth afterwards, anything that might change his mind.

He said awkwardly, 'I really have to go, get my passport from the top of Guillaume's fridge where it's been malingering since I got back from Cape Town.'

She stood there, in front of the broad glass window, the grey morning sky above her. The curtains hadn't been drawn. They had both fallen into bed at two that morning, him drunk and her exhausted, from an uncomfortable evening with some old friends of his from Oxford.

'Oh God,' she said in one breath, and then with an effort started moving around the bedroom looking for clean clothes to put on, avoiding his eyes and his body.

*In fact, you fucking little shit, you aren't coming back, are you? Am I right or am I right?*

At that moment two things leapt into her; that in ten minutes the apartment would be empty of him, and she would still be seeing his presence for weeks, until the image of their life blurred and dragged across the apartment into a few, probably one, convenient memory. And that she cared infuriated her pride, and instinctively she started turning his leaving into relief, explaining to herself it was a blessing she would no longer be involved with someone so immature. Neither of them said anything, and Wes finally picked up his case. His explanations remained unsaid, fermenting in the space he left.

*       *       *

Each day peeled back and revealed another raw part of Gwendolyn, and more changes in her body. Her breasts became weighted and the nipples darkened; things were becoming unfamiliar. What was most different, she told her friends, was the excitement. She had become stale, and London was stale; she felt people were pretending to love their lives and to understand England. Her friends didn't agree with her scorn, and asked her if she was having the baby for the right reasons. 'And what would they be?' she asked, but she knew they hadn't a clue either.

Now she purred to herself as she gently oiled her stomach every night before bed: 'I am going to have a baby. My own little world is about to have a population explosion. Someone is going to think I am the best thing since sliced bread until they are fourteen years old.

'By which time,' she fantasised, as she made herself another slice of toast of sardines and anchovies, 'I shall be different.'

Her father said, 'Come with me to Rome for three days. I'll pick you up tomorrow morning.'

One good thing about having no boyfriend is that lonely fathers take you under a wide grey wing again.

He had arranged to hear Valery Gergiev conduct the Santa Cecilia orchestra. With them was her father's second and favourite cousin Raphaella, and her boyfriend Otto, an elderly Austrian of thin character who seemed to Gwen to only enjoy his nearness to Raphaella, who affected not to notice him. Gwen thought he was vital to Raphaella though, a foil, and wished she could have a male handbag like that. As the dinner evolved, Raphaella, her dark eyes flashing, started arguing with Gwendolyn's father about collaborators during the Occupation. Gwendolyn knew that whatever side her father took, he was primarily inter-ested in baiting and sitting back to enjoy the spluttering and

Raphaella's desire to impress him with that peculiar feminine logic, which was something he valued and despised in equal measure.

Gwendolyn tried to seamlessly involve herself in their conversation, even tried to become interested in Otto, thinking that his views on wartime collaborations would be far more intriguing. But she felt herself floating away from them. The concert had been more intimate; like a tourniquet it had tightened the undigested emotions in her neck, she thought she would cry for ever, until the applause finished and she soaked her face with cold water in the Ladies' room.

'Got her hook into me,' he said as they wandered over a wide empty road the next day. Gwendolyn and her father were looking for a taxi to take them somewhere neither of them had decided to go. It was the November sun in Rome, a bright cold light on the bare, crumpled afternoon, and so they walked and he was talking as if to himself.

'What?' Gwendolyn said. 'What did you say?'

He pointed to the opening of a piazza, and they chose one of the uninhabited cafés that had spindly metal chairs outside.

'Got her hook into me,' he repeated. He opened his mouth and pointed down his throat, like a fish. 'Her hook went in so deep I could never get it out.'

Her father as a fish on the end of her mother's line, twisting and choking for thirty years. Gwendolyn thought about it, gingerly turning this latest explanation from this angle to that. No, she didn't believe in it at all. But he likes to think he does, she thought. He is moving from carriage to carriage of this story, wobbling along and wanting me to admire the same view.

He flickered his eyelids, and raised a thickened but elegant hand to the girl who now stood next to them holding a small menu. She was dark and seemed preoccupied, staring at a bit of a paving stone just beyond their table. Or perhaps she had bad eyesight and was wondering something about the ashtray. Gwendolyn had given up smoking for the pregnancy, so she recognised its allure.

'*Buon giorno*. Two beers, please.'

The waitress took a yellow cloth out of her apron and wiped their table, noticing Gwendolyn's belly with a slight and warm expression, before disappearing inside. Gwendolyn put on her new dark glasses.

'Now I can't see your eyes,' he said flirtatiously.

'Haven't you ever worn any?' She realised she had never seen him in a pair. They slowly discussed whether they were really necessary or a lazier way to hide your feelings, and that led on to a reluctant argument about global warming.

He was saying, 'Sun lotion, utter waste of time and money, all you need is vitamin C,' when he picked up the thread of the larger subject as if she had also only really been thinking about that too.

'I had such passion for her, and she was then beautiful beyond anything, but she was with Clive. We all used to go out to dinner. Great fun, Clive – they were two peas in a pod. Wild, always unfaithful to each other and always furious about it. Enormous personality, your mother.'

Gwendolyn was reminded how the word 'personality' had always been a horror to her. Behind it seemed to lurk toads and darkness. Those without blinkers were roadkill in the glare of a personality.

Because of the unexpected silence, the lack of apparent interest, he looked at his daughter, her hair curled into a chignon, her stomach leaning into her black dress, her scuffed trainers painted with neon markers, and her tights torn. Her strong chin he saw his own mother in, and her quick slanted blue eyes that always gave her away.

'But how was it when you both had us two babies,

within two years, and Laura being Clive's? Did you mind, was that the strain? Did she resent you, that you had a life apart, and she had to give hers up? Or did you resent her more? And how did you know I was yours?'

She kept her inflections playful, her tone even. To also say, I am not judging, it's all just interesting to me, that's all.

He looked a little startled, and his light brown eyes then filled with a sort of quizzical warmth she could feel.

'Your own smell to you in a way no one else's do.'

They drank their beers.

'Your mother wasn't ready for it, having children. Overnight became a monster, but the hook, you see' (and he opened his mouth in the same mime) 'was in too deep by then.'

They stood up and continued walking, and he took her hand in his and said, 'But I have you now. It was all so unavoidable. Life is, you see. I never divorced her because I loved her and my parents were divorced, and I believe it is a worse thing. You see, she couldn't help loving him, but she wanted, thought she needed, the security I could give her. And I, I was a moth to her flame.'

So he had known, the truth had just rolled away from him: he had been pushing it before him like a dung beetle all this time.

When she had finished packing, Gwendolyn suddenly remembered a conversation from when she was thirteen, with her mother in Jamaica. In the huge noon they were lying next to each other by a pool, Gwendolyn trying to look relaxed, and her mother naked and slathering coconut oil over her legs. She had asked her mother what her problem was – with Gwendolyn herself, anyway.

'Your birth was awful, went on for two days, and the disappointment was devastating. A boy was expected and wanted by both of us. I had been to an abortionist, and

163

changed my mind at the last minute. Before that I had sat in a hot bath drinking a bottle of gin, but you wouldn't budge. I thought I would be in and out of your father's life within a year, but after you I was trapped.'

Her mother with her tan and her wide smile, Gwendolyn's surprise and the silence between them for a while until they murmured to each other from under their sunhats about lunch.


Wes came back, shocked to hear she was having a baby and hadn't told him. He gave her his passport. 'You have my life now,' he said, 'you and it. I'm not going anywhere.'

He looked after her, and Gwendolyn gratefully accepted anything he did, let herself remember again the first time they met, the first time he proposed marriage after their third dinner together, told her quite sincerely that his girlfriend was casual, a bore; he had been planning to ditch her for a long time but felt lazy, now it was easy. That he had wanted her to get pregnant. But Gwendolyn now knew there was a subtext unavailable to her, that had provoked him to leave. Almost every day she felt the overwhelming fear it would pull him away again, and that she must keep as calm as if she were in a war, suspend any hysteria until the baby was safely born.

'I would rather you stayed,' she said as the last dredge of a stormy fight ebbed. Guillaume, his friend who had introduced them, Guillaume, who had assumed they would only last a few nights, Guillaume had now offered Wes a plump trip to the Yukon for *SmartTraveller* magazine.

'Last week's scan showed the placenta still hasn't moved up,' she told him. 'It's called *placenta privae* and I'll die bleeding within eight minutes if it bursts from the weight of the baby, and if this happens, the baby drowns immediately.'

But he had already gone; his eyes had the look of someone channel surfing. Gwendolyn watched herself for signs of revulsion, but the survival impulse was too strong.

On 2 April at three in the morning, Gwendolyn went into labour, a day before the planned Caesarean. She called a mini-cab and her sister Laura, who was in bed with a new boyfriend and said she was in Watford, but Joe had a scooter and if she couldn't get a cab would use that.

'Hang in there,' Laura said, 'I'm there.' But she sounded unthere and her voice was too loud and uneven. She's stoned, thought Gwendolyn, and apart from coming round to cook her dinner once, hadn't exactly been there for her in the three months since Wes had left. She won't get it together till morning.

Gwendolyn called her father, but his cellphone was off and she remembered he was in Montreal for a meeting anyway. She had packed her small case the night before, folding three tiny Babygros, an expensive cream shawl Laura had given her, her nightdress, underwear and sanitary towels, a hot-water bottle and disposables and two books she saw herself contentedly reading while breast-feeding. She was trying to think about anything else but what was about to happen. All she wanted was life, to be here tomorrow, with a baby in her arms. So please God, she was thinking, bring us safe to the hospital in this smelly dark Vauxhall Cavalier with the purple-turbaned driver who keeps looking at me in the mirror and who is taking us over the traffic bumps even though I told him not to.

She held her hands under her huge stomach, and tried to soften the jolts and not gag on the sickly Meadow Medley air freshener. She could smell the Number Six and onion bhajees. I will be all right, I will. The lights turned red. He seemed a nice man, this driver.

'Where's your husband?' He turned to her, smiling in the dark, not wanting to be cruel, but nevertheless it was an obvious thing that this pale blonde young woman had no one with her, not even another woman.

'Oh, he died, last month. Fell out of a window.'

The lie was her little triumph. If he had, she thought, how would she feel? Better. She wondered what it would be like to be this cabby's wife, probably leant on, spoilt, berated but totally secure. He would never piss off; men like him did not believe in the romance of the independent whatever, travelling through life as if they were in their own epic. No, they loosely inhabited a shared concept of God or something. Was he Hindu or Muslim? But whatever, his wife was bound to be safely swathed in material when she went shopping, secure her husband was mini-cabbing about London and not finding himself on top of a pack pony doing Fab Photos.

They arrived at the hospital, her driver paternally holding her arm, carrying her case into the reception. The bony nurse on duty behind the desk took her name and phoned her in to go upstairs. She had dark rings under her eyes, and quaint frosted orange lipstick. A brisk red-haired male nurse came across, picked up her case and led her to the elevator. How far apart are our lives, she thought, following him as he minced ahead. Pregnant women are probably repugnant to you. That's not fair, she reminded herself. How is he supposed to know how singularly weird such a commonplace thing as pregnancy is to most of us? Their shoes squeaked on the linoleum, and Gwendolyn noticed how each thing seemed clearer and louder to her.

'Please undress and put this robe on, and lie on the bed,' he said. A few minutes later, two nurses came in and were bright and chatty. They said, 'Oh, nothing to worry about. Now we'll take your blood pressure and temperature, put

166

this monitor around your stomach, to hear the baby's heartbeat.'

The room seemed too bright and too floral, newly painted. The tiny beats of him inside sounded like the beating of small wings against a window, a bee or moth or something, she thought. They left her alone. Someone had said – but who was it? – that three a.m. is the loneliest hour, the hour of grief. Think of something else, but it's four now, nearly. There would be a moment not far off now that she could disappear forever into. And if I am taken into the microdot of death I have the satisfaction of being more complete as I disappear.

Both nurses seemed impossibly important to her then, as they swept her down to the operating theatre like mothers in a Fairy Liquid commercial.

'Where is the doctor?' Gwendolyn asked.

'On his way. There's no traffic at this time of the morning – you've been very lucky,' Nurse One said.

Gwendolyn concentrated her thoughts into a holding pattern. Just let the doctor arrive safely, any doctor.

Nurse Two said, 'Would you like to be put out,' (like a cat, thought Gwendolyn) 'or do you want to be awake? The doctor has just arrived.'

She did seem so kind, this nurse, so Indian and clever, and so young too. She asked Gwendolyn gently again if she would prefer to be unconscious or awake.

'I don't know. Please, I want someone else, anyone, to make decisions for me for once. But, actually, I think I definitely want to be here, awake. Is that easy to do? I won't feel anything, will I? I definitely won't be paralysed for life?'

'Oh no, it will be fine. Right – we really have to do this now.' Nurse One went away and returned with Nurse Two, who was poised with a long needle.

'It will feel like a hard fist being pushed in,' she explained. 'Just try and relax. This is a spinal anaesthetic and works immediately, unlike the epidurals.'

Without more discussion they helped her sit up on the edge of the operating trolley and inserted the needle into her spine. The icy rush poured into her legs, filling her like a water jug.

Hands expertly slid her long frame on to her back, and she was wheeled in. Somehow the fact that it was the early hours of the morning made Gwendolyn aware of the background silence that would normally be filled with frantic hospital life, and she felt the cool dark outside present even under the quiet bright lights of the operating theatre. They put up a small screen in front of her face, and now the spinal injection had separated her body from her. I am only my head, only my breasts and my heart and my brain, she thought.

Gwendolyn realised she didn't know enough about anything – about who had made it possible over the last few decades for any sort of dangerous pregnancy to be saved. So that she, Gwendolyn Pound, who had only ever entertained fate as her one true faith, now owed life to this mysterious culture.

Dr Roberts was leaning over her, saying reassuring things. 'It will be over soon, stay calm,' he said as he walked the long way down, disappearing from view behind her tiny screen. Nurse One stood next to her, and held her hand. The doctor was cutting into her. An immediate falling away inside, her body knew it and she became faint.

'Give me oxygen, please,' she said calmly.

'Oh, you don't need it,' said Nurse One annoyingly. 'You'll do.'

'Yes I do, I'm going to faint. Now. Very soon.'

'If it makes you feel better then.'

The mask was put over her face and she thought, This is

unavoidable. I must remember to remember this. This was the bridge, this small moment staring at the ceiling keeping the mind here, this was the small time that was still just her, and he hadn't breathed his first, and they wouldn't yet recognise each other. She thought she heard the swoosh of blood falling into something, their heads seemed to stand back and then look up, and the firm and kindly Glaswegian Mr Roberts carried this bloody squirming baby to her.

'You have a son, Mrs Pound, a beautiful and perfect specimen. Well done.'

She gaped at the meandering fat limbs, the fat little face.

'My God,' she said. 'It, *he* looks like his father, after all this.'

She watched him being washed and weighed, fascinated, while the doctor and nurses involved themselves with sewing and closing her body up again, the body that had been briefly a swing door for her creation to enter her world.

Gwendolyn had changed, he saw that immediately he returned. He was languid with the brittle air of the Yukon still in his head, and the stale air of the airplane all over the rest of him. She looked tired and pale, but the way she was moving and meeting his eyes, he saw that somehow she looked older but better for it, and she was being too cheerful; it was definitely aggressive. The warmth he had brought with him fell and drowned.

'He's in there,' she gestured as she put the kettle on.

'How are you? I mean, how was it all? Did the birth go all right? Yes, it did – can I go and see him? You only told me a few bits and pieces over the phone, and you know I would have called more but it cost a bomb and it was someone else's.'

'Yes, it usually is someone else's. Despite and in spite of

you, everything went fine. It was a fascinating experience and I wish you had been there, but you couldn't be, so there we are. No point going over it now. What is important is you are here and Sylvester is in the spare room sleeping. I'm feeding him in ten minutes. If you want to stay, that's fine, if not that's great too. Really.'

Wes tried to make a pause in all this by looking out of the window, avoiding her glance. She was talking too fast, pointlessly wiping down the table, banging cups down and taking the wrong things in and out of the fridge.

'Look here, Gwen, I know I should maybe have come back sooner. I wanted to, I really did, we were so out of contact out there, it was wild. Really wild. I got bitten to death by mosquitoes, and it was fucking cold and our guide got us lost for a few days. We were scared, and I didn't even dare take my trousers off to have a shit because of these clouds of enormous mosquitoes. I mean, I am seriously constipated.'

Wes sat down slowly.

'But say what you have to,' he added. 'You deserve it. And I have jet lag, but anyway.'

'OK, let's clear the air for what it's worth. You have a lot of making up to do if you want to have access to your son. Right now, you do not get to pass Go, you do not get to collect two hundred pounds – in fact, you get jackshit for being nowhere when we almost died. I had to get a car alone and they did an emergency C section and no one was there for us – and don't get on that family thing again. You know my family only show up with flowers and disappear again until my funeral probably, more flowers, the Special Occasion Family, and yours weren't much cop either. They visited once and looked embarrassed. You are a fucking lowlife.'

She fell into the armchair. Wes was shaken, but not any more than she knew he expected. His mouth began to open, and she watched the speech slither down his neck from his brain till it moved his full and lovable but hateful mouth.

'Look, I do love you, Gwen. I've thought a lot about us and had a lot of time to do it in. The biggest space you could imagine, thousands of acres of trees and mountains and only Guillaume and the guide for company. And Guillaume met some girl called Alice in Vancouver, so that was him, and I felt ridiculous. Well, even when we went out, I was missing you, thinking of the mess I'd made. I was ashamed, I didn't know how to come back. I knew you'd be upset, I thought it would be best to leave it until the baby was born. I don't know much about that sort of thing, I'm sorry. I have, I *had* no idea how dangerous the pregnancy was.'

'The doctor did tell you. *I* told you.'

'Well, he hardly made it that clear I should stay, did he?'

'That's because he thought you were a hopeless case, and it would have been a waste of breath, which it was because I tried and you wouldn't listen.'

'It's not my fault he never told me. I would have stayed, of course I would. Anyway, as it was I had to get drunk every night to block out the pain.'

'Oh, poor you. Your whole life must be a miasma of pain then.'

Gwendolyn got up and he noticed for the first time she had cut her hair a bit, not much, maybe four inches but it was a start of something, or maybe an end. She returned with the sleeping tiny baby, wrapped tight in a pale blue shawl.

'Look, look at his tiny hands. He looks like you.'

During the times Sylvester slept, his soft, quick-breathed body lying in the crib, Gwendolyn would sit in her armchair with tea or a drink depending on her mood, staring at the television. She had this constant insane lightness, even as she threw objects at Wes – as if he was a coconut shy – it was there, the sensation of being a mother. Then there was the new father, cups of tea in the morning, love you, shall I take the baby, love you, just going to get the paper and yes, I love you too, can you switch off the light now and stop reading. It was a weaving in and out of overwhelming emotions for Gwendolyn, but being happy families was ballast, their courtesy to each other. And now the shared exhaustion became another bond.

One day, without particularly having planned such a move, Gwendolyn packed her suitcase and a bag for Sylvester. The sun came out that morning, after several weeks of downcast weather had started to drive people into sullenness from being trapped under a pasty sky and the damp-flannel air. Sylvester was now five months old, and Gwendolyn realised she was stronger.

She left on the M4, hailstones sliding down her windscreen, the wipers furiously adding to the drama. Sylvester drifted off in the back, his round gingered head rolling on his chest. She leaned half round and, while manoeuvring on to the motorway from the sliproad, pushed his head back and wiped his dribble with his blanket. After a while when the rain and hail had stopped and she was just engaged with the road, concerned only with the relaxing sort of worries like how much truth was there in the mythic white-van lore, whether the driver behind her was severely tired or just a woman-driver-hating bastard, she started singing, singing loud.

It was early afternoon when they arrived at Helen's bungalow, which squatted beside the busy road that cut through what had once been a village. It was comforting to be in this nostalgic geography of her early childhood. Built in the late sixties at the end of the garden of her great-grandparents'

Edwardian villa, it was cheaper than a divorce after forty years of shouting at each other. Her grandfather, Roy, died shortly after moving in, the peace and quiet too much for him. Now the house had been sold to a young professional couple, which meant they were tidy and commuting, leaving their two Persian cats to pad across the garden and over the wooden fence to the bungalow.

When Gwendolyn walked into the tiny hallway she smelt the trademark Gran smell of stale cigarette smoke and Vaseline Intensive Care hand cream. The nurse let her in; a dumpy lady in her sixties wearing alarmingly thick glasses that made her eyes bulge. She had only a slither of a kindly manner, but she smiled at the glamorous grand-daughter from London.

'Hello, I'm Rosemary. Oh, you've brought your baby all this way! Let's hope it's one of her good days. I'm sure she would enjoy her what, is it a girl? Oh, her great-grandson then.'

Helen was sitting in her only armchair, the dark red one, that Gwen remembered from childhood was the boat upon the raging sea of the living room, with the sofa being Laura's pirate's ship. The television was on, the sound down. It was rather small, and didn't have satellite. This annoyed Gwendolyn immediately, because she should have thought of organising that. And a proper cleaner, the dust was disgusting. Just these two women cooped up all day and night. Gwendolyn realised that she had to get some money together for vital luxuries.

'Hello dear, how wonderful to see you, and give your gran a hug.'

Gwendolyn put Sylvester on the floor, threw her arms around her grandmother's neck, rocking her gently, and wondered why it had taken so long for her to realise that they both needed this, this sort of love.

Rosemary stuck her head round the door.

'Do you need me for the next hour?' she asked. 'I thought I'd pop home to feed my two dogs, only they've been stuck in since six this morning.'

Christ, thought Gwendolyn, two other frustrated lives because of this cancer.

'Before I leave, I'd love to talk to you, Rosemary. I'll be going around nine tonight, or I might stay in the spare room, if it's made up.'

Rosemary's expression said, Yes, well, it's all right for you, farting about changing your mind, but some of us have to have a routine. And you with a baby.

'Right then, see you both in an hour.'

After rummaging about with a lot of key noises, she left, letting the front door bang shut.

'Oooer, you upset Rosie. You are naughty. Now what's that on the floor, is that your baby? Oh let me see!'

Gwendolyn carried Sylvester over and put him on Helen's lap. Helen laughed, 'Oh, he is wonderful, what a little character! Do you know, he reminds me of my father! That takes me back, my God. Forty years, is it – no, fifty or more – the way he looks at me with that smile, and the colour of his eyes exactly, that dark nut-brown hard stare. Just like my father.'

'What was my mother like then, as a baby?'

'God, I can't remember. Funny that, but you have to look at the photographs to remember your children, but parents stay with you, I suppose.'

'But what was she like? Growing up?'

'Oh darling, you know, full of it. Like this one here, but it's hard to tell at the moment, he's too young. She used to stay in bed when the doodlebugs came over, she wouldn't get out of bed for Hitler even – oh, she was a one, your mother. Look at his red hair! My, that must be from the father. Who is he anyhow? Don't you go marrying him if you don't want to, now!'

'Well, I don't know, Gran. I might have done a year ago, but he's been such an arsehole since I got pregnant. I mean, he's hardly around, or he is now, but only when it suits him. Shall I make tea, by the way?'

'Listen dear, you should know by now all men are selfish bastards. Look how I suffered all those years. Oh, you can't change human nature, and this is all that's important, right here. What a charmer. Are you giving him the tit, or the bottle?' Helen was looking into Sylvester's eyes and he had gripped on to her finger, which she was pulling up and down to his delight.

'Both,' Gwendolyn said. 'The bottle actually. Tried with the other, didn't work after a month, I was too exhausted.'

Gwendolyn decided she might as well stay, and made up the bed herself to make sure nasty nylon sheets weren't used. Despite being half out of it on morphine, Helen seemed fine enough to watch Sylvester, keeping him from rolling too near the electric fire with her foot. Laura had been the week before, bringing a huge bunch of yellow roses that were now starting to rot in their crystal vase. Gwendolyn was emptying it in the kitchen, when she heard a moan. She went back in, saw that Helen's face had drawn down in a sudden tiredness, and realised that her grandmother no longer recognised her.

'Oh, I'll give him his bath now, Gran,' she said, carrying her son to the sofa, 'as soon as Rosemary is back. How are you feeling? Should I be doing anything?'

'Where am I?' Helen said, looking wildly round. Sylvester began choking on a huge cry that was about to come out unless Gwendolyn fed him, now.

'Er, you're in your sitting room at Dandelion View.'

'Oh. And where's Roy?'

'Roy is dead.'

'Oh.'

Helen's face had lost her; she looked as if she was trying

175

to see in sudden dark. Gwendolyn had heard she could become like this, and just needed reassurance. Where the fuck was Rosemary? Sylvester was letting it rip, which didn't help Helen.

'Oh my God, what's that screaming? Oh, stop it, take it away! Where is my Roy? I want my Roy. Where is that bastard anyway?'

'Oh Christ, he's dead and buried.'

Helen looked shocked.

'Sorry, Gran. I mean – you know, he died years ago. Sorry.'

Gwendolyn took Sylvester out of the room and rocked him while she waited for the water to boil to heat up his bottle. She gave him a tour of the bungalow and the movement soothed him; his wailing had gaps now.

'And this is the spare room . . .' she said gently to him '. . . always cold as a witch's tit, and here is the bathroom, smelling of damp shagpile, and here is your great-granny's bedroom, the bed and the dressing-table with the thick deep scarlet grunge on a corner where my mother dropped her first bottle of nail varnish. Oh, look at this!' Gwendolyn picked up a small black-and-white photograph from beside the bed. 'It's my mother, on rollerskates holding Granny's hand on Brighton promenade. How happy they look. The forties, the war, rations and doodlebugs. Gran said she was a real minx. We'll go there next,' Gwendolyn whispered. 'Get some of that full briny air into us.'

A key struggled in the front door, and she heard Rosemary bustling in. 'Oh now, what's all this, Helen? Let's try and calm down. Bloody hell, I was only away for an hour.'

'I think,' said Gwendolyn imperiously, 'she should have had some morphine by now. Could you give it to her now? She is very distressed.'

Rosemary took her pastel-blue overcoat off. 'You just take care of that baby and I'll do your grandmother.'

The rest of the evening Gwendolyn just held on to Sylvester, letting him go to sleep in her arms, both of them wrapped in an old bed blanket. At nine she phoned the flat. The machine was on, which was a relief.

'Hi, we're at my grandmother's and staying here the night. Sylvester is asleep. I'll call sometime tomorrow.' She wanted to be able to say more, but wasn't quite sure what.

Wes was in the pub alone. He felt unwashed and confused. He thought about the whole thing, his son. Sylvester was focusing more, and he could see Wes at ten feet now. Before, he had been this blob really, breathing in a land of blur that was safely in his father's imagination. Wes reminded himself he was doing well for a man new to this all.

Usually he got on with life, sorting out his negatives and setting up jobs, getting drunk with friends. It was a weightless sort of pleasurable fear, this fatherhood, a long-drawn-out terror he must watch over. He listened to his thoughts spill over into each other. He'd have to be a hero for them, and he could hardly be one for himself. His father wandering about playing on the local bowls team at weekends, masons in the evening. His mother caught in a 1960s amber dream of her own, old-age New Age and wherever she went to inside herself, his father had forgotten how to retrieve her years ago. No, Wes had something to do in life, or the huge fanged dog Failure would be there, dribbling and panting over him.

The doors swung open and Guillaume walked in, looking cosmetically tousled and incredibly rested. It was already noon and time for a drink. He sat down opposite Wes on a stool.

Guillaume felt for him, man. Must be a tough call, he

177

told Wes, with a kid and a woman you weren't too sure about.

'Me now,' his eyes seemed to Wes to be laughing at him as he spoke '. . . me now – well, man, you know it's all about being free, being caught and that's sort of delicious, you know, like good dessert, but getting free again that's another rush, and that's men and girls, man. I love love too much to sit on it too long and get it dirty.'

They laughed without looking at each other.

'Maybe, you know, when I'm fifty, and I'll meet a woman of say twenty-five, or -eight, and she wants my kids, then I'll be ready for that. She'll think I'm brilliant and you know that's what we want, because let's face it we're vain fuckers at heart.'

They both went on like this, tossing the situation between them. Wes saw that Guillaume was now on the other side, the shore Wes didn't even know existed till he was off it. The pub was now wheezing with men standing at the bar jangling change in their pockets with guarded and grey smiles, and saying, What'll it be? There was a stale damp air in this pub that no amount of smoking and sweating would warm.

'Look, I'm off home then. I'll call you later,' Wes said. He waved weakly and sauntered out of the pub. He thought to himself, I am now a man with a woman and child, and I could swagger now, and also stride about. Twenty minutes later, after the scenic route, he reached Gwendolyn's flat.

Gwendolyn seemed to him to be less angry with him, and he thought that was very, very nice. In fact, despite the past, it could be just right. Goldilocks had finally eaten from the right bowl, and slept in the right-size bed. He picked up Sylvester, who smiled with a huge pink wet mouth and looked in the vague direction of his father's face. Wes put his nose between Sylvester's flopping head and shoulders, into his tiny neck – the best bit of a baby, full of their sweet smell – and kissed him and made eating noises.

'Do you think we should get a bigger place?' he said, turning his back so Gwendolyn couldn't see him smiling, and pointing out of the window to Sylvester at a plane grumbling away over the rooftops.

'I don't know. Probably. I have to wash my hair, and shave my legs and then one of us has to do the shopping for the weekend.' Gwendolyn paused, and knew Wes wanted to be looked after by them. 'Let's think about it anyway,' she said.

She went into the small bathroom, with all her bottles stuffed on the shelf, her bath full and scented as a secret empress's. She began pulling together the long trail of hair, twisting it into a rope around her head in front of the mirror. She said quietly to herself, 'I like holding his hand at night going to sleep, but not the pain of his casual cruelties.'

She looked herself in the eye. Someone had to take out the rubbish and wash up sometimes, to be part of this as well. She put a foot in the bath. How to grow another skin, she thought. That is one more thing I have to learn. She stretched her body out under the warm oily water and sighed, turning the hot tap on again with her foot. The door opened a bit, and Sylvester's small frame seemed to be walking through, held under his little arms by his daddy's long-fingered hands. Wes had that soft look in his eyes she only saw after sex. He knelt back in the doorway, putting the baby along his lap.

'Think about it while you're having your bath then,' he said.

# Taipei, Expectant

## *Bernard Cohen*

### (1) 18 November: Jetlag

My body disagrees with the physical evidence of time. Following the flight, I lie awake in bed. In this nightlit hotel room, our daughter's face appears to me like Chinese paper; my vision publishes unknown characters on her monochromatic forehead. I blink to clear it, but the ideograms persist in the gloom. My eyes, though still believing themselves subject to European clocks, have chosen an Asian insomniac alphabet.

Our daughter's folded-shut eyelids make crescent moons. She is two years old. Two and three-quarters.

We are in Taiwan, where I have taken up a short residency. This country invites me as a writer, and as I pass through Immigration Control I become illiterate. The streets are unreadable.

Nicola is six months' pregnant. Our second child presses legs and arms against the lining of the world.

'The baby will come after you are three,' we tell our daughter.

'I want it to come now,' she insists, as she has maintained for the last three months. Our daughter has no conception of a month. We explain that the baby has to grow more first, and that the exact time of arrival is beyond our control. She has known of parental fallibility for some time, at least since I proved unable to conjure her favourite television programme from a schedule of confessional talk-shows.

Our daughter wants her mother always, and refuses sleep until we are tired too, reminding us of the inescapability of parenthood. She wants reorganisation. At night I rest my hand on Nicola's belly and feel the thrust of a contained limb. 'Kick, kick,' Nicola comments. We are exhausted, having taken Oolong tea for hours.

That evening, I indicate to the stall-holder the fish we will eat, not knowing its name in any language. Our daughter asks for chicken. She can distinguish between chicken, which we eat, and 'real chickens' which run around and say 'buck-buck'. We do not know the source of our daughter's beliefs. Nicola and I back away from speaking of causation. I cannot pause outside restaurants where our daughter wishes to observe fishtanks as though they were aquariums. I put on myself the condition that if we were to stop and watch the fishes' oblivious trackmaking, I should have to explain to her the purpose of the tanks, point out the rows of diners behind.

At the table, someone compliments our daughter's cuteness, but in Japanese. I respond in my few words of Japanese, but the man continues in Chinese so the conversation ends. Why Japanese, I wonder, for speaking of cuteness?

I have developed interesting patterns, far from desirable. Unable to stay awake through our daughter's complaints that she is not tired, I collapse at nine p.m. for half an hour, and do not sleep again until four a.m. At midnight I go to my choice of two local Internet cafés: *Non-Mainstream Library*, with low, comfortably upholstered lounge chairs in private booths and very slow connections, or *Ezy-Cool.Net*, where dozens of teenagers play loud shooting games at every hour of the day, exclaiming across the room against a background of loud Sino-Pop. At the latter,

I am very old: a ten year old with a rasping voice screeches victoriously; I'm wondering where his parents are. I check obsessively for emails, but cannot remember from whom. I am waiting for something. I finish, and a bleached-hair youth tears himself from the game to charge me at the members' rate. I should be writing. This is the object of the residency. It is my job to write.

I am floating, or am failing to be grounded in a floating world. I feel as though I am between things. When should I wear a suit? Is it polite to offer whisky to young women? Was the taxi driver correct that one-third of Taiwanese have cancer? Did he mean that one-third of the population will die of cancer? How does it appear to locals when I attempt to conform to the rites of the exchange of cards? Polite? Ridiculous? Nonetheless, I give and receive with two hands.

I am an inadequate tourist, able to calculate the number of buildings I have seen, but not to recall their names. Nicola flies with a doctor's letter in her ticket wallet. Her pregnancy is progressing normally. No one reads the letter, possibly because Nicola's long coat disguises her shape.

In Taipei, we eat well, usually, by selecting a stall or cafeteria where we can point to the food we want. Our daughter refuses everything but noodles, and will only consent to eat noodles if we refer to it as 'pasta'. She asks for sandwiches and gets what she wants.

The baby kicks hard, visible through Nicola's stretched shirt.

## (2) 1 December: *The doctor doesn't know our secret*

Nicola has an appointment to see a general practitioner for a check-up and ultrasound. We all go, make it a family outing. The doctor, recommended by several expatriates, pronounces what he assumes we would be pleased to know.

'I can tell you,' he says, in answer to no question from us, 'looks like a little boy. Here is the scrotum.' He points to some grey on the screen. He is looking vicariously pleased.

This is not what was supposed to have happened, but I feel calm – no anger – about his spoiling of our surprise (or intensifying it if he's wrong). Over here, I don't mind believing that I know our baby's sex. I am transformed by the setting.

In England, the radiologist had made it clear that even if we were to ask, we would not be told. Her explanation: frequency of error. I wondered if the true reason was error or something else, the fear of other-cultural preferences for boys.

Later, I make the effort not to refer to Nicola's expanding belly as 'he'.

We do not give our daughter this new information. She will be a big sister, and she seems determined to be a big sister to all the world, but we do not specify a little brother.


*(3) 10 December: Collision*

In Taipei, I am waiting. I walk all day and observe a minor car accident under the expressway that runs above Civil or Civic (depending on which map) Boulevard. A taxi drives into the rear leftside of a businessman's car. Both drivers jump out to see what damage has been done. I am on the blind side. The accident strikes me as noteworthy because I am surprised it is the first I've seen. People drive in different patterns. My enlighteners explain that there are two road rules:

1. Fill all available space
2. Try not to have an accident

This is the sort of information that gives a visitor a sense of connection, of progress towards cultural comprehension.

Later in the residency I discover a third road rule: drivers must wear seatbelts on the expressway. The taxi drivers buckle themselves in as we enter, unbuckle as we exit. There are no belts in the back seat, and Nicola and I take turns wrestling our daughter still. This is another reminder that we are outside our lives: at home, we would not drive without the child's seat.

On further walks I see two other accidents, also minor. I cannot decide if this number over six weeks is statistically significant.

Lunch: hamburger, which I feel ashamed to have chosen. I am eating beef here in Taiwan, which I dare not eat in Europe. I'm told that cheap beef is Australian; more expensive is from Japan. For my own reasons (being Jewish), I don't eat pork, and in my notebook have sketched a pig's face to indicate what I wish to avoid. I show a stall-holder in a market, who grunts emphatically and with considerable porcine realism. We both laugh. We understand each other.

After lunch I return to the hotel, where our daughter bans me from speaking with Nicola. Nicola complains to her that we haven't seen each other all day, and I add my agreement as if this in itself would persuade. Eventually, I distract her with a present. She's in a good mood because Nicola has arranged for her to play with other children.

Nicola and I converse. It has been too hot, and Nicola is tired from walking. I am in a bad mood because I have written nothing, despite sitting over the keyboard most days. I promised my novel to the publisher months ago. (Despite this, our correspondence remains friendly, light.) I am trying to be conscious of Nicola's advanced pregnancy, to allow this to primarily inflect the residency, to explain my dislocation.

'Of your published books, which is your favourite?' a journalist asks, next day. My main duty on this residency seems to be speaking with journalists. Most have written several novels and up to half a dozen short-story collections. The newspapers here publish short stories. 'Is writing like giving birth? Do you think of your books as like children?'

'No,' I say. 'I can't forgive their faults.'

Journalism's funny. I've never understood it. Do I love my books? How could one imagine an assenting answer? I love our little daughter who wakes in the night and demands biscuits. I could not be an ideal interviewee because I do not talk about waiting for our second child in relation to my publisher's waiting for my novel. In my favour, I do not demand analogous answers of the tea-shop proprietor, cooking up her product in a flat (belly-like) wok. I also do not speak of our daughter's birth, how the labour began and ceased, began again. There is no relation between giving birth and writing a book.

Half-seriously, Nicola and I discuss our daughter's potential as product: advertising and the like. Our daughter has curly hair and a luminous complexion. Wherever we go in this city, people ask permission to photograph her. We refer the requests to our daughter, who invariably refuses. Her admirers are surprised, but accepting. None attempts surreptitious photography. Similarly, I do not attempt to take photographs in the National Palace Museum, nor in the National History Museum where one hundred and twenty ancient, life-size terracotta warriors have been loaned by Mainland China. I would not use a flash – my camera is old and is not even equipped with flash – but the rule is firm.

Nicola and I have evolved roles: I buy meals from the stalls, and she does grocery shopping. This was not consciously worked out, but our daughter immediately identifies task with parent, wants to accompany me to the 'café' and Nicola to the supermarket. We do our laundry in the bathtub, and overheat the bathroom overnight to dry our wrung-out clothes.

## (4) 15 December: Various games

Shaving rash dots a line around my throat, though the water here seems much less irritating for my skin than that in London. Our daughter stands beside me on an upturned wastepaper bin, and shaves with a soapy piece of cardboard. In most of her games she casts herself as the Big Sister. Her doll is the baby.

She asks: 'When the baby comes, Daddy, will you bite it?'

I explain that we don't bite people, that biting is not a good thing to do, but that I will comfort the baby when he or she cries and look after the baby as I do her. Our daughter seems dissatisfied.

At night at the Chiang Kai Shek Memorial, soldiers armed with dummy weapons practise disco parading to Western show tunes ('Tequila'!). Our daughter dances across the steps. The weather has been fine, hardly a drop of rain.

When it rains, I gather our evening meal on my own. The scents around the food stalls concentrate; there is no longer a general food ambience, but specific aromatic pockets by food region or type. I feel proud of this observation, and tell a journalist, but it appears in the report as 'fruit' rather than 'food': eccentric rather than insightful.

Our daughter wants bedtime stories about what the baby will be like when it comes home, stories demonstrating that Nicola's and my love for her will not diminish. Her grandmother has sent a book on jealousy, and she wants us to explain how one gets it. Jealousy sounds interesting. We promise that the baby will not try to take her toys immediately on arrival. Looking into the future, I think I can foresee occasional difficulties.

## (5) 29 December: Departure

Each movement towards leaving is delayed by one step; the steps are cumulative. We shop too long for last-minute souvenirs, and our daughter (who has been sleeping in her stroller/pushchair) wakes, will not stop crying. Nicola is trying on clothes. We imagine these clothes fitting less than two months in the future, when she will become less bulbous.

We return to the hotel to finish packing. We cannot fit all our possessions into the suitcases, all our daughter's new toys. I go searching for a cheap sports bag, but have left it too late and cannot find one.

A car arrives to take us to the airport. Our daughter is impatient to return home. The baby wakes and squirms, and Nicola places her hands on her belly. At the airport, we discover our flight has been cancelled. We are sent to the old terminal by shuttle bus, our journey rescheduled. A new friend, a Taiwanese academic, comes to see us off. I joke that the new terminal is just a set, that no flights have ever left from there, all are cancelled and rescheduled. We spend the last of our New Taiwanese Dollars on a toasted cheese sandwich for our daughter.

Goodbye, goodbye.

At Hong Kong International, I buy Scotch, we eat cold chips, our daughter loses her temper. Fourteen hours later, at Heathrow, the jetty fails in the icy weather, and we must wait an extra forty minutes to emerge into England, blinking.

# East of the Mountains (extract)

## David Guterson

Beneath stars, as in a dream – Emilio before him, Sanchez at his back – Ben stumbled through pines and into an orchard where the dark apples had not yet been picked, on between rows of silent trees, until he emerged in a dusty field. The lights of a dozen trailer homes burned; pickers stood about. The place seemed blurred, but flat and still, as in a photograph.

They hurried past the first three trailers, where pickers gawked like spectators at a race, men and women standing in the cold, their hands stuffed in their coat pockets, their hats pulled low on their foreheads. It was clear that few were abed in the camp, dogs wandered in agitation, children ran footloose and dumbfounded in the night, their faces tired, quizzical. Emilio ran through without stopping to speak, without apology or explanation, and the pickers moved to make room for him and for the strange-looking doctor with one eye swollen shut, wearing steel-rimmed spectacles, his boots untied, limping. Emilio pressed on toward a silver trailer hulking in the dark like a dry-docked submarine or airplane fuselage. Its low door was thrown open, and a woman waited there, in vigil.

As they approached, she clasped her hands beneath her chin. She was fat and wore a parka patched with duct tape. 'You are the doctor?' she asked.

'Let us through,' said Sanchez.

'Thanks to our God,' the woman said. 'I have been praying for you.'

'Let us through,' repeated Sanchez.

Ben put his head in the trailer door. The room had the feel of a cave or chamber; distorted shadows shimmered against walls of riveted, contoured aluminium. The spectral light of a kerosene lantern illuminated a macabre scene. At one end of the trailer, on a bare mattress thrown there as if by a tornado, a woman – a girl – was in the throes of labour, naked and twisting on a nest of blankets, bucking and swaying on her hands and knees, her eyes shut, her belly heaving. Her hair had matted to her shining face, obscuring half of it. She tucked her head between her breasts and groaned until the cords in her neck bulged; then she fell on to the lengths of her forearms and paused to catch her breath. Her feet kicked spasmodically, she cradled her head in the palms of her hands, her face lay against the rough mattress. She rolled on her side, flailing, and a wail escaped from her lips.

A young man in stocking feet knelt beside her, brushing the hair from her cheek with his fingernails. A woman knelt on the mattress, too, speaking urgently in Spanish. A second woman, short and large – a dwarf, Ben realised: she was four feet tall – stood with rolled sleeves at a propane stove, dipping a towel into a kettle of steaming water, then wringing it with muscular vigour. 'It's good you're here,' she said to Ben.

'How long has she been in labour?'

'A long time. Too long,' said the dwarf.

Ben ducked inside, carefully. The ceiling loomed claustrophobically low, and he couldn't stand without stooping deeply, which hurt his neck and back. He moved closer, knelt beside the mattress. The girl, he saw, was very young, a child giving birth to a child. 'What's your name?' he asked.

'Her name is Doris,' the boy answered, and draped a blanket over her.

'How old?'

'Fifteen.'

'Are you the father?'

The boy nodded.

'What's your name?'

'Jimmy Perez.'

'This is her first?'

'Her first, yes.'

'OK,' said Ben.

The woman on the mattress caressed the girl's damp forehead. She seemed to Ben to have an eye of glass, or a wandering, unfocused, dead pupil – he couldn't tell which. He couldn't tell if she was looking at him. She seemed to look sideways, or through him, or beyond. 'Are you her mother?' he asked.

'No,' said the woman, her eye roaming.

'How long have you been here?'

'I came last night.'

'Twenty-four hours?'

'More than that.'

'She's been in labour twenty-four hours?'

'Longer,' said the woman.

Ben shook his head. 'Are you a midwife?'

'I don't know anything,' the woman answered.

Ben put a hand to his forehead, pausing. He had not attended a woman in labour since his internship in obstetrics forty-four years earlier. For six weeks in 1954 he'd assisted in delivering babies. 'We need to call for an ambulance,' he said. 'She needs to go to a hospital.'

As if in response, Doris heaved painfully on to her back, seized the hands of the glass-eyed woman, and bore down with so much force, her lips whitened, her eyes squeezed shut, tears leaked from their corners. She flung her legs wide unabashedly – a seething mass of dark tissue, her purple rectum swollen. The vulva had stretched to the limit; her perineum might rupture. An episiotomy would have helped, but that was impossible now.

'Can you do anything?' asked the glass-eyed woman. 'What are you supposed to do?'

Ben didn't answer. He kept his hand on his forehead. The girl panted, gasped, and grunted, then bore down again. Ben saw the swelling of the baby's head, the wet, dark oval of its hair. 'The head is showing,' he said.

'What does that mean?' asked Jimmy.

'It means it's too late for the hospital.' Ben turned to the propane stove. 'How hot is that water?' he asked.

'It's too hot,' the dwarf said. 'I'll put some cold in it.'

Ben took off his hunting coat and rolled up his shirt-sleeves. The dwarf poured dish soap into his hands, and he washed, adjusted his glasses on his face, and knelt again by the girl. 'You're all right,' he said.

'Are you a doctor?'

'Do I look like one?'

'No,' said Doris.

'Well, I am.'

As if in answer, she pulled at her thighs to spread them as wide as possible. Then she buried her chin against her chest and bore down with the concentrated force of a woman trying to move the earth. Her skin went from grey to blue, her brow furrowed, her eyes narrowed; it appeared as though she was being crushed by something enormous and invisible. Ben watched while the baby's head crowned, and then Doris's perineum ruptured. There was blood now, but not very much. The tear looked relatively superficial, involved the fourchette and mucus membrane but not the underlying fascia. 'Your baby's coming,' said Ben.

The dark wet head emerged gradually. It came face down, then turned sideways – a natural restitution. The features were scrunched, constricted, crabbed, the eyes clenched, the mouth closed, the skin tinted a shade of blue far darker than the blood of veins. The head stopped, came no farther, and seemed to retract or shrink again, like the head of a turtle or snail. An odd, swollen, parasitical growth attached to the girl's groin. Her gaping legs with a head between them – a neckless, embryonic head. It hung suspended, a third appendage, Doris impaled on it. Ben lay on the floor beside the mattress to wipe its strictured face with a towel and swab its mouth with his forefinger. He wished he had an aspirating syringe, and even more, a fetoscope. The baby wasn't breathing, it was stuck at the shoulders. He wasn't sure what to do about it, but he knew there was no time to lose. The cord might be fatally compressed.

Ben pulled up Doris's left knee until it pressed against her swollen belly, and then he brought up the right. Doris held them there. Awkwardly, low against the mattress, he pried hard at the baby's head, stretching the neck unnaturally, then gave up and slid two fingers in, next to the baby's ear. Doris shrieked and swore at him in Spanish, and Jimmy Perez put a hand on her back and leaned close to her. Ben was relieved to find that the umbilicus wasn't tangled, but he still felt time was running out. He slid in a third finger and tried to twist the baby, turn it in some subtle fashion, unlock it as though the passage to birth were a Chinese puzzle of sorts. He tried clockwise and counterclockwise. He couldn't think what else to do. He withdrew his fingers and pressed on the girl's pubis, as though the baby might be popped free, as in a Heimlich manoeuvre. It didn't work, and he pried again, gripping it behind the ears. The baby remained intractable. 'Is it dead?' asked Jimmy Perez.

'No,' said Ben. 'We'll get it out.'

'Its face is blue.'

'It isn't breathing yet.'

'It's dead,' said Jimmy.

'No, it isn't,' said Ben. 'It's still getting blood from the umbilical cord. That blue will go away.'

'It's dead,' said Jimmy. 'I know it.'

'No,' Ben repeated.

He slid his fingers past the baby's neck – slid them into Doris's vagina. He knew he was hurting her – she was trying to pull away and shrieked at him in Spanish – but he had no choice any more. His hand was in, now, to the third set of knuckles. Doris winced, holding her breath; her face blanched, her eyes closed. Ben crouched with his fingers inside her, seeking with his fingertips. He followed the length of the baby's upper arm, which was folded across its collarbones, until he came to the little elbow. It took a while. He searched. Finally he found what he was looking for. When he drew out his hand, he had the baby's small blue fist trapped between two of his fingers, as in a magic trick.

The baby's arm hung quivering near its head while Ben popped the shoulder free in a gradual release of traction. The other shoulder came much more easily, and the baby – a girl – slid out like a fish, awash in blood and amniotic fluid, the umbilicus wrapped around her. 'You have a new baby,' announced Ben.

Catching her, he trembled. He held her, a jewel, in his palms. 'It's a girl,' he said. 'She's beautiful.'

'A girl,' said Jimmy Perez.

'Thank God you were here,' exclaimed the glass-eyed woman, her pupil crackling with light.

'Let me,' said Doris. 'Let me see her.'

Ben ran a finger inside the baby's mouth, then blew in her face to startle her. Next he turned her upside down, his hand locked around her ankles, flicked the bottoms of her feet gently, then slapped her on the back. The girl began to wriggle in his grasp and made small squawking noises. She turned pink gradually. When she started to cry, her father crossed himself. 'A miracle,' he said.

Ben was still trembling. With a towel he swabbed the baby clean, then set her, covered, on Doris's belly. Jimmy lay down to look at his daughter. He covered his mouth in disbelief.

'What do you need?' the dwarf asked.

'A sharp knife,' said Ben. 'And some twine.'

Sanchez, from the doorway, produced a lock-back blade. Ben sterilised it in rubbing alcohol brought from a neighbouring trailer. Then he tied the umbilicus in two places, using bits of manila twine, and made his cut between them. The placenta delivered of its own accord. Ben made sure it was all there, then dropped it into a plastic bag the dwarf held open for him. He washed and looked again at the child, who was nursing vigorously. Her colour was substantially better now. She had a lot of dark hair, and a cowlick.

Ben pressed gently on Doris's lower belly, assessing the condition of her uterus. It was hard to the touch and had contracted swiftly to the size of a small grapefruit. She was not bleeding, and he felt satisfied that there was no immediate danger. 'You should take them both to see a doctor,' he said, addressing Jimmy Perez. 'After she's rested, but as soon as possible. Just to make sure every-thing's all right. That there aren't any problems.'

'OK,' said Jimmy. 'Thank you.'

'There should be a clinic in Wenatchee,' said Ben. 'They'll have a doctor who knows about this, who knows about newborn babies. And someone for Doris. She needs stitches.'

'OK,' said Jimmy. 'We'll go.'

'It's dangerous not to,' Ben warned.

When he went outside, it was first light. The orchards nearby were hung with ripe apples. The broad sky was pale, cloudless. Things looked different now.

# Rosemary

## Kathy Page

You're a girl, though I don't know it yet. Another thing I don't know is who *I* am. For most of my thirty-eight-year life I've not wanted you; then I realised that I did, and thought it would be impossible. Now, I can scarcely believe how easy it has been, nor how much you have altered me. Breasts, belly, heart, lungs, the pigmentation of my skin, the volume of my blood – of course, but this goes way beyond the physical. You've unpicked my vigilance, turned me all of a sudden into someone absent, dreamy, squeamish, alternately fierce and vulnerable. I'm even less objective than I was before. I shouldn't be giving other people advice. But that has occurred to me far too late, so here I am – along with you, of course, greased, furry, eavesdropping, hiccuping, somersaulting and thumb-sucking inside – not what I was, not quite what I will be. I am giving tutorials and running very late.

Rosemary is the last student of the afternoon. She's a short woman of perhaps sixty-five, once petite, I'd say from her hands, but now short and plump. She's wearing beige elasticated slacks, and a cream-coloured blouse, not tucked in. Her hair is scooped into a loose grey bun, her skin crêped with age but still noticeably fine and soft. Her eyes are a clear, pale blue but there's nothing jewel-like or penetrating about them. Like everything about her they seem gentle and blurred, as if the colour has been achieved by some kind of washing and fading process, over many years. She smiles, just a twitch, as she sits down beside me at the huge refectory table. Opposite is too far away; this way we have to twist to see each other but can read the text together.

'Rosemary –'

'How are you, dear?' she says at the same time. 'It must be hard work, this . . . in your condition.' Her hands lie loosely, one on each thigh. She wears a thin wedding ring, nothing else. I'm staring too much, I think, and make myself glance away, out beyond the shade of the room at the garden, the hillside and the sky burning blue with summer's first heat. Then I come back to the room. Rosemary's two neatly typed pages are on the table between us, next to each other. Most people write reams. It's unusual to be able to see an entire piece at once like this.

'I like it,' I tell her, 'though it is very short. I'm not quite sure about the way you end, and that's mainly what we should talk about. Otherwise there's not much I think you need to add, or take away. It's very vivid, and clear that the child has been betrayed, and of course, that she can't tell her aunt. You've done a good job.'

'Good,' Rosemary says, leaning back a little, patting a loose strand of hair back into place. 'You see, I did live with my aunt. It's all true.'

'Ah,' I mumble, unimpressed, because *all true* tends to mean *I won't change a thing*; it makes for a more difficult and much longer session, and I'm already very tired and increasingly aware of your foot in my ribs and an ache, high up in my back, from sitting so long here at this table, necessarily further back than is comfortable for reading.

'This incident is part of a longer story,' Rosemary explains. 'It's not supposed to be a story on its own. So I didn't want to make it end properly because I've done other bits that come later.' She smiles, then adds wistfully, 'Such a strange family, we were.'

And at this point, she waits, looking straight at me, for some kind of reply. And if I were my proper, professional self, I would protect both of us by talking about the problems and blessings of using autobiographical material, the questions it raises, the ways it can be used as a springboard for fictional ideas. I'd be asking: 'What is your aim with this piece of work? How long will it be? Have you got a sense of the structure?' But as it is, I run my eyes over Rosemary's face, meet the pale blue eyes (mine are similar, but newer) and let them lead me astray.

I ask: 'How, strange?' I'm busy, flexing my shoulders, stretching my neck, feeling you take up new positions in the spaces I've made and I just don't think where this might lead. Though thankfully, given what she says next, I know it's not the sense of a voice you recognise, just the *sound*. And Rosemary's voice is as brisk and bright as a waitress announcing today's special.

'The thing is,' she tells me, 'my mother's father had been through one war, and couldn't bear the thought of another one, so he shot himself –' she pauses a moment '– and then, once he was gone, my mother, poor woman, tried to kill herself too, many times, in most ways you can think of . . .' This too feels like a pause, not an ending. And while I'm not keen on all this suicide, something, perhaps Rosemary's face (it attracts me; I'd like to touch it, to test the softness that I see against my own skin), encourages me to trust that there will be something good the other side of it. So I wait, my attention shifting between her and you, and the window. It's another new thing: these days, I find I can more easily wait.

'Then, of course,' she says, 'as well as that, my mother tried to kill me and my brother. Twice, that I remember. I was six, he was four.' She taps the paper between us with her forefinger, the skin pale and freckled, the nail neatly filed, French polished. 'That was just before this happened; it's why we had to go and live with our aunt, you see.'

'Your mother tried to kill you? How?' I wish immediately that I had not asked, because I don't really want to know. In the past I might have, but these days I have to close my eyes when blood is spilled in the cinema. I, who once wrote with relative ease of a variety of horrors, including infanticide, who invented diseases – as if there weren't already enough! – find cruelty of any kind both more difficult and more painful to imagine than I used to, and cruelty to children impossible, even though I know it is real. And as for tragedy, I push it right away! I refuse to know, as if that might make it go away. I want shadows banished, loose ends tied; I long for resolution. I want the world to be better, fast – so that you, the space traveller coming slowly to earth, will be safe all your life.

'Oh,' Rosemary says softly, 'this is turning into some sort of confessional, which I really didn't mean to happen.' But all the same, she smiles her soft crinkly smile and goes on with it. And my swollen heart beats harder, in case I have to do something: extricate myself, fight her, shout, run . . .

'I'm going backwards from the end and I haven't written this bit yet,' she says. 'The poor woman couldn't cope. War again, and she thought that the German tanks were going to come rolling over the hill so she'd better save us from them and whatever they might do. It unhinged her. The first time, she tried to gas us, along with herself, of course. We got away because she passed out first. But the very next day she cut our wrists. I climbed on a cupboard and managed to get out through a window to a neighbour's house, and again we were saved. My mother was sectioned, and, as I've said, we went to live with my aunt.'

Rosemary calmly unbuttons the cuff of her blouse for me to see the scar, thin and white now, almost innocent in appearance.

'It's a terrible story,' I say. It is, it strikes me as I speak, the story of a mother who could not bear the thought of tragedy, and longed for resolution.

'They're very neat scars,' I say. All that suffering squeezed into such small marks.

Though actually, there's more.

'Until I had my daughter,' Rosemary says, 'I didn't truly understand my mother. But after Susanna was born I was in a dreadful state; I often wanted to kill myself. These days you'd be prescribed a tablet to sort you out, but then, they didn't even have a name for depression. So I pitted myself against it. I lived. The idea of the suffering of others, of my little girl later in her life – that kept me from suicide. So I understood my mother then. I forgave her. Maybe she was not quite so strong as I was, perhaps she had more to bear. Really, she was a gentle woman; she meant no harm. It was a perverted form of love.'

This must be the end, and I am grateful for it. To make certain, I name it.

'You broke the pattern,' I say. 'You stopped it from repeating. You made something else happen instead.'

'My dear,' Rosemary tells me, leaning back. She pulls her cuff down but leaves it unbuttoned. 'My dear, I only had the one child. And she is forty now, married to a lovely man. They are very happy as they are and have decided they definitely won't be having any children. Let me tell you, when Susanna told me that, I wanted to cry for relief! It's really over now, I thought. Everyone is safe. Now everything will be all right. I believe that. I know it will, and that's why I want to write it all down – though somehow,' she adds, 'it's harder than I thought . . .'

How dare you, I think, the flesh tightening on my arms, my stomach suddenly hard as the stretched muscles pull tight, practising for birth, *how dare you* tell me such a sad and terrible story? Your mother tried to kill you, and your

daughter killed her children before they even existed –
what kind of ending is that?

Naturally, if I were able to be my proper, professional
self, I'd be saying, 'Isn't this a wonderful example of the
way meaning is construed according to our pre-existing
ideas. Doesn't it just show how everything is a matter of
interpretation . . .'

For a moment I'm too angry to actually say anything at
all. Then I look across at Rosemary smiling back at me
with her clear gaze and her hands loose in her lap, and
everything melts. I know for sure that she too is a gentle
woman, who means no harm. She is sitting next to me on
the wooden bench, but at the same time, she is still inside
the story she's told. She's in an old-fashioned kitchen that
smells more every minute of gas, reaching above her head
for a door handle that's just out of reach. She does get out.
But the very next day it's going to happen all over again, in
a different way . . .

Rosemary gathers her papers and slips them into a file,
the file into a plastic bag.

'I'm so glad you liked it. And good luck with . . .' she
adds, and gestures uncertainly at where you are. And then
she's gone.

I have been no use at all.

However to make a happy ending out of this?

I sit alone for a while in the shadowy room, close my eyes
and wait, sunk down in myself so low that I can feel the
slightest thing. As happens occasionally, you've fallen still,
and I want you to come back. For a long time, nothing
comes. Just the sounds of others in the house and garden,
the smells of food being prepared, my own breath going in
and out. Then, at last, a muddle of movements comes all at
once, some kind of impossible gymnastics, an origami of
flesh. Elated, I stand and make my way to the stairs; climb
slowly to my room. And with each tread that's left behind, I

forget Rosemary's terrible story a little more, until it has shrunk to a tiny nothing at the back of my head to be written as 'Rosemary' underlined twice in the margin of my notebook. I'm doing it for both of us. I'm doing it for both of us, because this is how we must go: muffled, blinkered and blind, empty of knowledge, deaf to warnings and ignorant of history . . . you and I, the two of us, moving on but also going back to where everyone has been before. Everything will be all right.

# Looking for Sylvia

## *Kathryn Heyman*

Downstairs, a kitchen is opening for business. Pots bang, forming a percussive bass-line to the murmur of voices. Someone empties a bucket outside and two women call to each other, their words drowned by the rush of water. Martin is still snoring beside me, mouth parted gently so that his chin forms a double lump. The hotel clock clicks over one more minute: six forty-five a.m. Since five, I've been lying here, watching the numbers change. Click, click, click, while I lift my legs in the air, up and down, trying to get rid of the nagging cramp travelling along my shins. I pull the sheet back and look at my naked belly. A ripple runs over it as the baby adjusts position, its feet settling up under my ribs so that any breath is squeezed out and a little more acid is squeezed in. Martin gives a loud snort as I push myself up to sitting and waddle, teddy-like, into the small, pink ensuite.

Pregnancy, in the late stages, is supposed to make women bloom. Your hair grows glossier, your lips fuller, your skin clearer. Except for me, apparently. My hair is half-matted, my eyes red from lack of sleep, my skin patched and mottled. It is true, though, that my lips look full and red. I pout at myself in the mirror, then say, 'Mummy.' It feels silly, but I try again: 'Hello, I'm your mummy. Your mother.'

Then I remember Martin, all motherless and alone. I sit on the closed toilet seat, put my hand on my bump and whisper, 'I will always protect you. I will. I promise.' Even as I say it, I'm filled with fear, thinking of Martin's mother, the mother who could not protect him. I should say: *I will try to always protect you. I will try to live for ever*, but it doesn't sound good enough somehow. Not by a long shot.

The bump moves and I feel a slight trickle leaking out on to the lid of the toilet seat. That's the other thing: no bladder control. Eau de urine, for the blooming woman.

Martin lets out a loud groan. He often moans in his sleep. Sounds of real distress, which I always put down to his mother. In the mornings, I tell him that he was thrashing about and moaning. I usually add, 'It's grief, isn't it? For your mum.'

No, he says. He slept like that long before she died and it is too much cheese or wine or not enough sex or just a bad dream – and why does everything have to be about his mother anyway? I say nothing then, keep my lips in a tight little line. Because it seems so obvious to me. Everything *is* about his mother.

I go back into the bedroom and stand looking at him. In some ways he does look like a child, his mouth open, spit dribbling, face soft. There's a photo of him at the funeral. Why would you take photos at a funeral? No one does that, do they? Someone took this, though, of little Martin. Square, black-rimmed glasses, huge on his tiny face, like the too-big suit dangling off his body. Blond hair poking up as if he's just got out of bed. And his eyes, staring through the camera, all blank, as if he can't remember his name. I found it when we moved back to London. It was tucked into the back of *Three Kittens in a Boat* and when I tried to show it to Martin, he pushed the photo back into my hand and said, 'Oh, *Three Kittens*, I used to love that story.'

She used to read it to him, acting out the parts of the kittens. That's what his father told me. There's a photo of her reading to him. You can't see what the book is, whether it's *Three Kittens* or not. She's blonde, too, like him. Same thin, brown nose, same smattering of freckles. There aren't many photos of her later, when she got sick. Martin says she was bones, just bones.

When I stand up to clamber into the shower, another trickle seeps down my leg. I wipe myself again, with the quilted toilet paper, but there's more by the time I get back to the shower. At the ante-natal classes, they said there would be a show first. The midwife said we didn't need to worry, we'd know when we were in labour, and we'd get this red or pink in our panties. She looked all pink herself when she said *panties*. I decide it must be wee, because I don't feel anything: no desire to nest, no tightening anywhere, nothing. Anyway, I haven't come all this way to go back without even getting to see her grave.

By the time I get out of the shower, all red and blotchy, there's more liquid and I smell of musk. Like sex. Not that I'm getting even a little bit of that at the moment. I get heartburn or cramps every time I move, so jiggling up and down on top of Martin hasn't been appealing for a good few weeks. I stick a wad of toilet paper in my knickers and pull my hair back so tightly that my eyes go all almond-shaped. Although I used a loofah in the shower, I scrub at my back and legs with the rough towel. I want to be clean for her. More liquid seeps into the toilet paper and slowly, slowly, a little door opens in my head, lets a chunk of light in. Screwing up my eyes, I concentrate on the liquid coming out of me. Thick and mucous, I know it isn't wee.

I know what it is, or at least I have half a clue. Martin has scrawled the number for the local hospital above the phone, just in case. He's been anxious the whole trip, waiting for contractions, checking every day: *Do we need to find a doctor? No?* It was my idea, I thought it would take my mind off waiting. Everyone says the last two weeks are the worst, just sitting around, checking the calendar, and fielding phone calls. *No, nothing yet. Yes, we'll keep you posted. Yes, just waiting.* My sister, Becky, told me no one comes early. Not the first time. Her first three were ten days late, the fourth on time and the fifth, Ginny, with her crooked little walk, came twelve weeks early. Only just viable. I've read all the books, I know the terms, and I know this too: my sister nearly didn't make it back. For all the talk of how easy labour is these days, it's still going to the brink, still terrifying, still death-defying. When it comes right down to it, past my belly oils and Active Birth classes, past my endless reading about Gestation and Dilation and Immunisation, past all of that, down deeper than my womb, what I get to is this: absolute terror. I will come back different or not at all. Now, with the musky liquid seeping out of me I realise that I don't want to go on this journey at all. I don't want to go through with it. This comes to me with a supreme brightness, so crisp and clear that I want to sing.

Last night, when we got to the hotel, Martin and I sat outside in the dark, whispering. I held his hand, asking what he remembered. His voice was flat, the way it is when he doesn't want to go on, when he wants me to just shut up. Nothing much, he said, nothing much at all. Only these things: her hand striking him across the legs in a supermarket; her voice telling him that she did indeed know best; and her body doubled over like a rusted paperclip, carving out six-foot letters on Harlech Beach. I AM NOT GOING TO DIE. It took her all afternoon and she kept at it long after her two boys and their father had given up and gone up the hill to the café. They sat in the conservatory, watching her down on the beach hunched over her letters with desperate concentration. I AM NOT

GOING TO DIE. A message of terrible hope to her children, their breath steaming up the glass of the window. When she finished, she stood up and waved her arms at them. Like little sticks, Martin said, ready to blow away.

When he finished giving me his little memory list, he got out of the car and slammed the door. I sat in the dark, sobbing.

Later, in bed, after we'd counted the horse-shoes printed on the wallpaper, he said he remembered coming here, looking for Sylvia's grave. He was still in a pushchair. He said it as if she'd committed a crime, dragging a child around a cemetery. That was the word he used: *dragging*. Even though if he was in a pushchair, it's obvious that she was doing the pushing, and carting all his weight.

He rolled over and said, 'I don't know why we're here, why I went along with it. You're just as obsessed as my mother was.'

'Actually,' I said, 'if we were obsessed, we wouldn't have to look for Sylvia; we'd know exactly where she was.'

When I first met Martin, he'd tell me his mother was a saint, a wonder. Years of me ranting in his ear, all my bullshit therapy-talk about how he'd painted his childhood all rosy and peach, how his mother was obviously controlling and self-obsessed, and suddenly she and I are allies. Us and We. Against him and his father and the world. Years of hating the hold she had on him, and now I rush to defend her, want to slap his hand if he raises it against her memory.

'She did the best she could,' I say.

'How she must have loved you,' I say.

Martin is still sleeping when I creep out of the door. Nothing rouses him, nothing moves him.

*     *     *

Cobbles stretch up the hill in a wet, dark line. Sylvia did not live here. She did not love it here or even, as far as I know, like it here. I slip on the cobbles, and feel a sudden surge of wetness slip down my leg. Wet toilet paper is glugging against my leg, but I am not coming this far for nothing. I will not leave without a photo, or at least a moment alone with Sylvia's grave. Martin doesn't know, can't remember whether she got to see the grave or not. Or whether she gave up and went home. Stupid, ungrateful man, forgetting so many of the details. I ask him: did she like to cook Italian dishes? No, this he can't remember. Did she find Morecombe and Wise overrated? No, this he can't remember. Once, just once, when I first knew him, he said, 'Maybe I'm angry with my mum for leaving. Mothers aren't supposed to die.' Then he laughed and ordered another drink. This is what he does: orders more drinks, changes the subject.

There's a man hosing the path down outside the cemetery and I stop to ask him where Sylvia's grave is. He looks at my bump, and then at my face. I don't know what he sees there, but he says, 'Should you be out looking for dead people in your state?'

A sharp knife slices across my spine as he speaks, and I grab hold of his hand. He seems terrified and starts backing away, looking over his shoulder, muttering words like *doctor* and *ambulance*.

My hand wraps around his wrist and I am surprised to discover that I am shouting. 'No. I don't need a doctor. Just tell me where it is.'

I take a breath. The pain has gone now and I feel calm, clearer and saner than I've ever been. Seeing the panic on the man's face, I try to exude serenity. 'Really, I'm fine. I've got weeks to go.' My voice is lower, less feverish, but when I laugh, I sound like a hyena on methadone.

Still shaking his head, he points to the back of the cemetery, where the weeds seem to sprawl. He grunts, 'Up the back. Don't trip on the stones, love.' His voice is thoroughly Home Counties, so I'm sure he throws the 'love' in to give me a taste of Real Yorkshire.

It surprises me, the easy way he points the grave out, as if he's been waiting for me to ask, as if he visits it every day. The lack of difficulty detracts from something. After all she went through, I should at least have to scout around, hunt her down. Surely it shouldn't be this way, every Clare, Tamsin or Sara knowing the exact longitude and latitude of her grave. It demeans it somehow. Demeans me. Makes it more like a visit to Graceland than a private pilgrimage.

A small, moss-covered step leads up to a gate into the back section of the cemetery. Just as I swing open the gate, that knife cuts across my back again. Then turns around and slices across the deep muscles of my abdomen. My knuckles stick out, turning white as I squeeze the hard metal. Deep breath. Eyes closed. After the pain goes, I hold on to the gate for a minute longer, looking at the brown puddle near my feet. Braxton Hicks. Must be. Because I am not ready, I do not want to go to that place. I just do not want to.

Before Martin's mother died, she was a woman with cancer, a mother with cancer. Before that, she was a mother. Before that, she was a woman who climbed rockfaces for a hobby, who taught her all-thumbs husband how to sail a catamaran and prune a grapevine. Before she was Martin's mother, she had a name. Dion. This is what his father told me: the day that Dion was told about the cancer, about the thing eating away at her insides, she threw a glass paperweight at the lady doctor, shrieking that she would beat this bloody prick of a thing because she was not going to die, she was never going to die, she would not leave her children alone, not for the life of her. Foolishly, she added: 'I will beat this if it kills me.' Martin's father thought there was a nice bit of irony there. Apparently she also used the F-word, and was escorted out of the surgery by a white-haired male GP. The lady doctor went home early.

What can you do, once you have a child, except stay alive for the rest of your life? What I mean, of course, is the rest of the child's life. And what about those who die in childbirth? *It still happens*. There's no reason in the entire universe why I should be one of the lucky ones. Leaving my child motherless, hopeless. Stumbling along line after line after line of scrubby-looking graves, I find myself praying, or uttering a kind of prayer at least. Oh God, I am saying. Oh God, oh God, oh God. Suddenly the pain hits again, like someone is digging into my bones, shovelling into my marrow, and I grab on to a tall headstone for support. Two dark-haired women pass me, arm-in-arm, like sisters. They look at me, doubled over the headstone, and ask if I'm OK.

'Fine,' I tell them. 'I'm looking for Sylvia's grave. Been here for, oh, must be hours.'

'Oh,' they say, sniffing the air.

They must have loads of us down here, really. Swarms of youngish women with gloomy faces and small handbags; just big enough for a slim paperback and a pocket camera. It must drive the villagers mad, the traipsing tourists with a penchant for death. At least, I can imagine that's how they see it. But it isn't that way, not for me. It isn't the oven or the poetry that gets me, it's the milk. That one small act. She must have been in a mania, that's what the downstairs neighbour said. She was on the stairs, her hair flying about her face, her hands waving around like wasps. Upstairs, the children slept, hearing nothing. And then, the details, as familiar as fairytales. In madness, despair, rage, jealousy, or just utter exhaustion, she switched on the gas, stuck her head in, breathed deep. But not before she taped up the door, ever so carefully, and left out a bowl of bread and milk. For the children, who would wake in the morning alone.

After the sniffy women move on, another wave of pain comes over. I let go of the headstone and walk up the long line of graves, my head turning, turtle-like, left and right. Names flash past: *Beatrice, so dearly loved*; *Andrew Colby, peace at last*; *Dora, our angel*. I'm moving fast, concentrating hard. And then it comes again and this time I can feel my insides opening up, making way; I can hear the trumpets blasting out the arrival tune. There's an endless list of names, but no Sylvia. Another slice across my back; this time so sudden that my mouth opens and a bit of a scream comes out. Count them, count the time between them, I remember that, but I have no idea what it's supposed to mean. It's all supposed to take hours, days. Count. How many seconds equals danger? Anyway, I have no watch, so I count in headstones. I get to the end of the row and turn up to the next one, scanning left-right-left. Eight graves between attacks. At the end of that row there's still no Sylvia. At the end of the third row I'm up to a knife-slice every three headstones and everything is pushing down inside me, pulling me down. I bend over a stone angel and vomit on its chipped toes, watching the streaks of orange and green dribbling down on to the grass. Vomit is on my trainers and I can see blood in it, I swear it's blood, and even though I still haven't seen Sylvia's grave, I start yelling. The words I yell don't make any sense to me, I think perhaps it's another language, one I don't know yet; but the dark-haired women hear and understand. Understand enough, at least, to run back and stand either side of me, rubbing my back, saying there-there. One takes out a mobile and – is she younger? Her eyes are darker and skin smoother and *ooooooooooooooooooooo*OHGODOHGODOHGOD

I disappear and reappear, and the two women half walk me, half carry me, out through the gates and down the cobbled street. It all looks so regular, so like it did an hour ago, except for the strange light hanging about everything. Catching the street at an angle, it makes things shine and refract so it seems as if they aren't quite real. Or aren't as real as THAT PAIN. There is a door, there are some steps. Some noise, something crashing. A door opens; I am in a room. There is some wallpaper, covered with horse-shoes. Someone calls to me, rubbing my arm. 'Who are you?' I say. It is the woman, the smooth-skinned woman. 'The ambulance will be here soon,' she says. Turns away from me, to someone else, saying, 'It's OK, she'll be fine, shall we wait?' Martin says, 'No, it's OK.'

How did Martin get here, into this room? His face is all turned in on itself, caved-in and red-rimmed with worry. 'Where is Sylvia?' I say. He doesn't answer. Instead, he rubs my arm, my back, my forehead. He is as annoying as a fly. I want no one now, I want no noise, I want nothing. I am breathing, very loud. There is me and my breath and the pain the pain the pain and that is all. Martin is somewhere, waiting. He will wait. I am opening, I can feel it, can feel my whole self turning liquid as hot silver. Some pounding, somewhere, and the door opens. Some-one has my shoulders; I think it is a woman, a paramedic. She puts a thermometer in my ear, pokes my arm, moves me about and lies me down. Ten centimetres, she says, no time to get to hospital. I sit up, clear again. Martin moves over to me, pats my hand.

'Excuse me,' I say, 'I need to go to the toilet.'

The woman looks nervous, asks, 'What do you want to do?'

'Use the toilet,' I say.

'Bowels?'

'Sorry?'

'Do you want to use your bowels?'

It comes fast, urgent. I push at the woman and at Martin. I yell, 'I am going to SHIT.'

'Just do it here,' she says. 'Push, go on, push.'

And so I do. I squat on the floor and I push, knowing that there will be shit covering the floor but thinking, Oh, what the hell, you know? What the fucking hell. I push, feeling the shove across my back and in my bowels and then, feeling the shift, feeling the push happen in the centre of me so that I know I will split in two. The paramedic woman calls out, 'It's crowning, it's crowning,' and I put my hand down and feel a round curve of soft wet hair and I push and I push and then there is a wet wet slippery slide, the woman calling out, 'It's born, it's born,' and Martin crying and saying, 'Thank you, thank you, thank you,' and I put my arms down for the warm wet length of the baby and it's OK, I know it's OK, I don't even have to promise.

I am not going to die, not me. I am never going to die.

# Tales of the Recent Past
## *Nikki Gemmell*

*conception*

We have made love in the afternoon in Paris and T. has come inside me and it has uncoiled something between us. It is the first time someone has come inside me since I was a foolish teenager, and it has eradicated all the grimy sexual tension that has been there for so long, a couple of years now. After it I am nuzzling and giggling like a newlywed because I have come to a decision, the most magnificent, surely, in all of life – to renew it.

T. does not know of this. I have told him I am now on the pill. He is younger than me, and not ready for children. I do not know if he ever will be. But for me, time is running out.

I loop my legs above my head, tall into the air. My toes touch the wall behind me, spilling the sperm down.

'You make happiness come,' T. says to me during dinner. What will he say with a baby between us?

*one month*

I see babies everywhere, pushchairs, pregnant bellies, slings. A man at a party tells me he travels the length of London to smell a newborn's head. It is the most powerful, non-erotic human experience, he tells me, it is pancakes and vanilla and skin.

I read in the newspaper an article by Germaine Greer, saying that with motherhood, women willingly endure a catastrophic decline in their quality of life. I read a scrap from Sylvia Plath's journal, that she could be more imprisoned as an older, tense, cynical career girl than as a richly creative wife and mother who is always growing intellectually.

I do not know the effect a child will have on me. I have heard the horror stories: how it will be difficult to go to the toilet with a baby, or have a shower, or wash the dishes, or write a book. How a child saps your looks, especially a girl. How making love after having a baby is like throwing a sausage down the Channel Tunnel.

I am a little afraid. All I know is that my life will now swing like an ocean liner changing its course.

Five weeks after we have made love in Paris I vomit into the toilet, beside T., brushing his teeth. The next day, in a London café, I am so nauseous after a sip of water that I think I will have to rush on to the pavement and vomit into the gutter.

I can feel something drawing on my energy in a way I haven't been drawn upon before.

I haven't yet told T.

Two stripes on the white stick from the chemist. So, confirmed.

Hello, my little one, stomach-tucked, firm in the world.

*two months*

Today, seven weeks old, you make me vomit on the pavement outside the library and there is no time even for the gutter, and like a dog with its posts I am marking my haunts. But it's joyous vomiting, if there can be such a thing, for it is telling me that you are strong within me, that you will not fall away.

I have a craving for fresh meat and vegetables and ice and fruit. You drag me from my ruby wines and limpid cheeses, my peanut butter and pâtés. You've made me lose my taste for chocolate, you canny thing.

And now we are three. But T. doesn't know this yet.


*three months*

You are darkening my nipples, making them silky, widening them. You are lengthening my pubic hair, greying it. You are splashing my skin with pigment; there are spots on my face and hands, and a stripe that is bold down my stomach.

I push T. away. I don't want him now.

And still I vomit, sometimes so violently that I bring up clots of blood like small foetuses themselves.

And one day, one weekend, when I can no longer keep the vomiting a secret, I tell T. He crosses his arms and rocks back on his heels, like a spectator watching a Sunday afternoon cricket match. He enquires, casually, about an abortion. I have had two already. I tell him time is slipping away for me. He doesn't say he'll leave. He's younger than me.

He stops rocking on his heels. He says OK, OK, whatever I want.

Deep in that night we joke about what music you'll like and what your accent will be and your name. All we can settle on is Grain.

I have heard of men who vomit in sympathy with their partners. There is none of that with T., although he has a craving for hot dogs. We laugh a lot. I feel so fortunate. What could be more lonely than having a child by yourself in hospital?

And as I tell people of your presence I am enveloped by their joy, and I know now that I'm sharing you with a much wider circle than just your father and myself.

Old hands offer advice: see as many old mates as I can during pregnancy, use disposable nappies because life is too short, don't fight sleep, chant silently in labour 'My vagina is a slippery dip', that it actually feels like you are doing a very big poo, that there is nothing elegant about it and I am laughing and laughing so much.

But still I vomit, up to twelve times a day, especially when tired. On weekends T. holds back my hair from my face as I crouch over the toilet bowl, and swishes out the bucket by the bed and puts his head to my stomach and tells you not to make Mummy sick and I have never loved him more.

You will be a Chinese whisper of us both.

*four months*

You are turning me from my favourite radio station. I can't bear the dance-beat thumps any more, you're pulling me back to Bach, you're evening me, slowing me.

What will become of me now I'm a mother? Will I quit the arena of action and become a spectator in life? Will I live by reflected happiness now? It is the way of old people, isn't it? And mothers. I always had a secret disdain for them, those disappearing women, weak, faded, blended. Now I have a disdain for what I was.

My mother tells me I will shed all my selfishness when I am a mother. She tells me that having a child will settle me.

At night, there is the three of us with my tummy pressed into T.'s lower back and you between us and our breathing. When T. puts his hand on my belly a calmness blooms through me. He worries for you as I bend, and when my tummy fills with laughter which is often.

He hasn't told his parents yet. Soon, he says, soon.

I am rattled that I will have just a midwife at the birth in England and no one else. This overstretched country, I think. It is the twenty-first century and yet it feels like the days of Thomas Hardy. The hospital is on London's outskirts; it is grimly Victorian with windows grubby and tall.

Yet there is a wave of well-being that drowns everything else. Happy hormones, I read. I love my happy hormones, why can't they be with me always? They are skimming me through this pregnancy.

At the first scan T. and I are giggling so much you keep on veering wildly from the screen. But then there you are, back, with your little pod-hands and your quickening arm and your strange, fierce face when you stare at us. Tears at this confirmation: no, I'm not making you up.

But when will I feel you, little astronaut? When will you flutter in my tummy? It is almost eighteen weeks now and I'm impatient with your stillness. You are still dragging me into that deep, deep tired where I wake up tired and never find a firm footing with the day. Will it ever pass? Will I ever feel normal again?

Will I ever be alone again?

Will I ever feel so lonesome again that it almost hurts?

More, says my mother. For there is nothing like the pain of the love that a mother can feel for a child, especially when that child chooses to reject them.

But what of a parent rejecting a child, I wonder?

*five months*

Oh flutterer. I can feel you now, tummy-tucked. There are little seismic tremors and I laugh out loud. Ripple baby, tumbling and scrabbling.

You are changing me, making my genitals fulsome, ripe, plumped and I feel sexy and womanly and yet push T. away. My own body is enough for now, the wonder of it, it is all I want.

A sudden jolt against my hand – you prodder, you! – and T. hurries across but you won't oblige a second time. A mind of your own, already.

T. puts his hand on my tummy and it spreads calm through you, I'm sure.

Our love is knitting.

## six months

Being driven through France by a girlfriend and thinking of you incubating inside me as I prop my bare feet on the dashboard and laugh with my friend, Tam. Thinking of the times in my life when I've been most free, invariably alone, when I've been vivid and edged and aware. Can I ever have that life again? Tam laughs and says of course, I can just take the baby with me.

But an anchoring now.

You're like a little kitten with a ball of wool in there. My stomach is public now, hands reach to it often. I could spend hours lying in bed with my palm resting on my stomach, laughing. I wake in the night to T.'s laughter, to his hand on my tummy. How I love you so fiercely, already. T. whispers into my sleep that I'm going to make a lovely mummy and I smile in my dreaming.

Isn't such happiness obscene in one person?

It all seems so wondrous, and fresh, and unique. And yet this is so many women's story.

Relief at passing twenty-six weeks. You are viable now, such a technical term for such a wonderful concept. You can survive without me.

## seven months

In a couple of months I will never again control my life with the tight fist I have always been used to. I will have to surrender to the will of someone else. A child will drag me into life. I could be distant, remote, without one. As a parent I have to participate.

Growing heavy from you, cow-slow. Big now, waddling. Big face, arms, thighs. I have swelled from a D to a G cup and there is no bra that is sexy or even black in that size. Losing confidence. Becoming less me, more generic pregnant woman. Sharp, this loss of esteem.

Will you sap ambition? Will I be diminished? Made invisible?

T. tells me to chill, or you will come out as tight and curled as a tin-foil ball.

It is hot now, midsummer, and you squirm in my stomach. I have always loved the heat, now I don't. You are changing me so much.

You don't like me working, I can sense that. You yawl and tug when I sit at the computer. It is as if you are saying, 'Hey, swing your focus back to me.'

T. puts his wide, cool palm on my belly and instantly you calm. The rumpling stills, as if you are listening to his skin.

He tells us he has to go away.

An overseas commission, the most important of his career.

He'll be back in time for the birth.

He stands. He rocks back on his heels.

I ask him that night if he's ever smelt a baby's head. He tells me not to be ridiculous. Why would he ever do that?

I have never felt more alone in my life.


*eight months*

Busy at the computer because I have to be now, and in the thick of it you punch your fist up and I yelp at my desk. It feels that you will break through my skin, it's stretched so thin. Before, it felt you were cosy-snug in there, that nothing could get to you. Now at my desk I look down and there's a lump protruding to the left of my navel, a little head. Gently, I push it back.

I have not heard from T. He is in another hemisphere. I have no number, no address. He said he'd let me know.

And so I work. There is little time for panic. There is much to do. I have heard the word 'layette' for the first time in my life.

I put my hand under my belly, I cradle you in my arm, I sing you into stillness.

A shortness of breath now, even reaching for a plate in the cupboard. Blood swishing in my head. Sometimes you hurt now, getting a heel or hand caught. The hospital has put me on an iron supplement and my stools are hard and as black as ink. I am tired. I no longer laugh.

The midwife tells me your head is down and you are ready to come out. I ring T.'s family, leave a message on their machine, tell them it's urgent but no one rings back. So, he hasn't told them.

This is my choice.

I read in *Vogue* that a girl baby steals a mother's beauty. I read in *Vogue* that a boy baby makes a woman appear more masculine because of all the male hormones flooding into her body. I feel old from you, you are sapping me.

You are my choice.


*nine months*

Can I get any bigger?

Can skin stretch that far?

You push and jab with your fists and I can feel, sharply now, the wanting out. You wriggle when I write, for some reason – is it urging me on? Ssssh, it's coming, not long now. I'm speeding, little one, the overnight bag is packed, the toenails painted, the legs shaved. You're in position, head down, with your spine obediently to the left, you're readying yourself for out.

I can sense it, soon, and I am resting, nesting, like a she-wolf retreating to the hills. I am sleeping sixteen hours a day. The flat is spotless, clothes are washed and folded.

I can feel some urge that is old and wild and howling deep in me, something buried over many years, something subsumed by ambition, and work, and contentment.

## due date

Today is the day the computer has said you are most likely to be born. But you don't want to come, you're not ready. You've found a comfortable position in there, locking your heel on my rib and you don't want to budge. I can feel that my body is saying, 'Wait, rest, gather strength.' It's too tired at the moment. I surrender. I wait.

In the night there is a rippling across my tummy, below the navel, like a roll of thunder across the desert that amounts to nothing but signals a possible storm.

Then nothing.

For a week, nothing.

Just occasional Braxton Hicks contractions like a rolling pin over uneven dough, tightening around you and falling away.

I have not heard from T. I no longer ring his family. I have another focus now.

I try everything to nudge you out. Champagne and nipple tweaking and pineapple and raspberry leaf tea. Everything but sex.

*birth*

Awoken at three a.m. by what feels like a small, grey cloud drifting across my abdomen, as if a giant – or God – is squeezing my belly. Five hours later, ten minutes after my waters have broken, you are out, like a fish whooshing along a deck. Just gas and air to get me through it, just the midwife and myself in the birthing room. 'A textbook birth,' says the midwife afterwards, gently. 'An easy labour,' says my mother to her friends. I tell her that no labour is easy, that there was a moment during it when I felt like I was splitting apart, that there was a point where I said to myself, very calmly, 'I am never doing this again.' I had never imagined such pain.

I did not know I would defecate during labour. I did not know there would be so much blood. I did not know that for several hours after the birth my belly would resemble a child's attempt at baking a cake, all sunken and soft in the middle.

I did not know such love.

*now*

I write this in ten-minute bursts, once a day – it is all you will allow me. I sit at my computer in that wonderfully clear, bright, curious time in the morning when your day hasn't been corrupted by nappy changes and wind and too little sleep.

Six weeks after your birth. Flowers still filling the flat, just, blousing out, tumbling petals. Still bleeding, just. Still smell meaty and fleshy down there. My stomach muscle has split. A line of pigment still dissects it. My breasts have ballooned and dropped, they are marbled with blue veins like river lines on a map. When I urinate it feels ragged and loose. None of this matters.

Such love.

Your face is unfolding. Your ears are like two little squashed roses. Your hair, smoothed, is a shell-spiral; ruffled, a corrugated lake. Your tiny nails are soft and ragged until I peel them away, your hands balletic in sleep. Your eyes are deep and blank and dark and seem to go on for ever. Do you see me? I don't know. You see my voice, I know that.

I am exhausted. I am transfixed.

You are soaked in my fingers, nails, skin, clothes, sheets, hair. I have never known another body so intimately. The smell of your sour, milky breath, the palms of your hands, the powdery folds of your groin. We sleep as close as lovers, my arm around you, face to face, and my nipples drip watery, blue-white milk. Sometimes I think that you are cold, that all I am is a feeding machine, that I will soon be discarded and my confidence is shot.

But then you smile.

I have found a kind of peace with you, especially when I am feeding. You have forced me to be still, to distil my life. I have shed all that is extraneous because, simply, there is no time any more for so much.

T. has rung five times. I have never picked up the phone to him, never interrupted his message.

I can't stop smelling your head. And I have found another spot, the lovely, soft dip at the back of your skull, by your neck. It is pure, concentrated baby.

I am overwhelmed by the crush of love surrounding you. It is ferocious, this rush of joy, this tenderness of friends and strangers surrounding a newborn. 'God bless the little one,' says a waiter at a restaurant as we leave, and it fills my heart.

I am not afraid of us alone.

# The True Body

*Simone Lazaroo*

My mother Rose's pregnant body looks like a red sail full of wind. She steers it past the workshops full of heavy wooden Chinese coffins buttressed at their base like tree roots, past the gaudy paper funeral decorations which bluff and flutter in the breeze. Such weight, such lightness as she walks towards Sago Lane, where the dying houses for the Chinese are.

The crickets ascend the notes of their noon song until the pre-monsoonal air is shrill with it. It is a sunny afternoon in Singapore, 1960, more than fifteen years since the Japanese soldiers startled the crickets into silence and hung corpses from the lamp-posts, yet it is difficult for her to be sure on this morning which is the most imminent, birth or death. She is there, against the orders of her mother-in-law and the Malay midwife, to visit her old amah Ah Lai, the servant from Shanghai who wetnursed her when her own mother died during childbirth.

That morning, the midwife told Rose to put aside extra danger money for her. 'If you want me to deliver after you take such risk, lah! Visiting dying houses in the final days of first pregnancy, ah-yah!'

There is Rose then, disobeying orders, not even thinking about where she'll find the extra danger money, following her belly and her nose past the steam-filled laundry to the chartreuse-tiled Kopi Shop. She buys two squares of bright green-and-white striped kueh here. She swallows one in

225

two bites, feels it fold and wobble like a jellyfish as it slides sweetly down her throat. She carries the other in its waxed paper bag for Ah Lai.

On the corner is another Chinese funeral decoration shop, where the proprietor paints a stern red mouth on the face of a papier-mâché Zen Sheng, or True Body.

'Going to a Cheena funeral, ciap cheng woman?' he calls. The Chinese have called Rose's family ciap cheng, meaning mixed-up salad, for generations. Ciap cheng, after a warm salad made of both sweet and savoury ingredients. It's to do with the confusion of European and Asian genes in their blood. Rose doesn't blink at the insult, but the baby turns inside her.

The man keeps his eyes on the stern red mouth emerging from his brush. 'True Bodies ver-ree important for Cheena funerals. They give the dead person's spirit somewhere to go.'

Rose wonders if she could perhaps do with a True Body for herself as she turns the corner into Sago Lane. She feels detached from the heaviness of her limbs and belly, as if she is floating, or out of her body. She is only dimly aware of the turning in her womb as she comes to the entrance of the women's dying house. Such weight, such lightness.

The proprietor of the dying house is sitting on a chair out at the front of the building, picking at his teeth with a sharpened match. He has a mouth full of gold fillings and a chest full of gold chains above his impeccably white singlet. All this gold glints in the sun that falls between the dying houses. Rose wonders how much of Ah Lai's life savings this man wears in his teeth and chains.

She gathers her red skirt into a loose bundle around her belly. 'Ah Lai?'

'Down the hall and first turn left,' the proprietor says, immediately resuming picking at his teeth.

Rose passes a low table bearing spirit tablets, flickering

lanterns and little offerings of food for the dying house's recently dead. She walks slowly down the whitewashed cloister to her amah's room. She pauses at the doorway to draw sharp breath at the darkness of the long narrow room lined on both sides with beds, at the odour of urine and perspiration.

There are about twenty-six beds. Near the entrance of the room, one old woman is crouched upright on the edge of her bed, her long-nailed toes curled around its polished wooden rail like bird's claws. She nods almost imperceptibly to Rose as she passes.

In the centre of every other bed is a bundle of rags. Somewhere in each bundle of rags is a body, limbs, a wrinkled face shrunk by dehydration and age beneath a smooth, almost bald scalp. Most of the old women are still. Some of them pick with their thin fingers at flaky skin, or rub at old scars on stumpy limbs. Some of the old women's eyes are closed. Some of them are open, huge with unspoken suffering. Rose can hardly bear to look, but she has to carefully search each bundle for Ah Lai's face.

Near the end of the row is an old woman breathing like an animal in terrible pain: *huh huh huh*. It is Ah Lai. Her eyes are closed, but there are tears streaming from their corners and running into the grey wisps of hair at the sides of her face. Ah Lai opens her eyes when Rose touches her on her hand, but her gaze shows no recognition and her tears do not stop.

'Ah Lai, it's me, Rose. You remember Rose.' Nothing. 'I have brought you kueh. The green coconut jelly one you like.' Not even a flicker of recognition in the tea-brown eyes. 'I have a baby in my belly, Ah Lai.' The desperation of this motherless mother-to-be, bribing her wetnurse on her deathbed for blessings.

Ah Lai closes her eyes. There are tears, still.

All Rose can do is put the kueh down on the floor and

gather her old amah in her bundle of rags against the bundle in her own belly. Rose can't feel or hear her sobbing, but the wet patch on her shoulder from Ah Lai's tears spreads from a bud into a continent whose borders keep expanding across Rose's red bodice. She goes on holding Ah Lai like this as she watches the small tunnels of sunlight lengthen through the narrow windows.

The noise of the traffic builds gradually outside. It must be nearly evening when Rose feels an emphatic kick in her belly that sends an acute, itching cramp into her vagina. She puts Ah Lai down hastily on her bed and stands.

There is a warm gush of liquid which floods her thin lawn underpants and drips, then runs until a small pool forms around the wrapped kueh underneath her on the floor. She dips her forefinger into the little pool and tastes salt, ants and almonds on it. Rose feels as if she might implode into the pain in her belly, and yet she feels so far away from it.

She does not have the words for this. She pants: *huh huh huh*.

Ah Lai is panting too. Her vision flickering with each exhalation, Rose grips the foot of the bed and looks at her old wetnurse's closed eyes. In this breathing, in this roaring of air and this dimming of vision, they enter the long trembling opening of life, the long trembling squeeze of death.

'Ah Lai?' Rose whispers.

*Huh huh huh.*

There is only this from the bundle of life waiting for departure. This fight to breathe, which sounds like the wings of spirits flying towards their True Bodies.

There is another pain sharper and hotter than lightning, a flash of white and gold as the dying-house proprietor steps up, picking his teeth, counting his money, graceless angel.

\*     \*     \*

228

My mother Rose lies in the oncology ward of St John of God Hospital, a long red scar on her belly where her womb once was. She is fresh from the operating theatre, still wearing the hospital's green robe. Her face is as pale as a plate of milk above the green.

We do not know the test results. We don't know if she will live or die. All I know is her smile, invoking mine. She coughs thinly, her throat raw from the anaesthetic tube. It hurts her to speak. She closes her eyes.

Her breath is quiet and short: *hph, hph*.

Outside it is a spring evening in Perth, Australia, fifteen years before the close of the century. The sea breeze parts the veils of cirrus in the pale mauve sky. On the city streets vendors sell daffodils for the cancer foundation. I give them all the small change I have in my purse. On this evening, I hope for good more than I believe in it.

I drive with my husband to the fast-food hall of Myer Grace Brothers' department store, which is fluorescent, overlit. I at least have the words for it when my amniotic fluid floods the cake crumbs on the white tiled floor.

'My waters have broken!' I yell to my husband, who is perusing condiments at the far counter. The young blonde shop assistant freezes, her blue Wettex sponge held midair. Almost immediately there is a long, sharp pain high in my vagina. It is the direst pain. I grip the handle of the cool drinks fridge and breathe: *huh huh huh*. I drop the can of chrysanthemum tea clattering on to the glass counter and abandon my pool of amniotic fluid on the fast-food hall's white tiles. Looking back at the amniotic fluid, I see it's a small thing, not the flood it seemed. It is the first sign of the arrival of something beyond me yet part of me, something divine. It looks vulnerable, in the way the divine often does. I want to bottle it, or at least wave it goodbye. The Myer Grace Brothers angel descends upon it with her blue Wettex as my husband guides me to the lift.

I know my statistics before and during pregnancy. 35–24–34, 40–46–36. I know how to time contractions. Twelve and a half minutes apart. I know my True Body, it seems.

In the car the contractions escalate to six minutes between each one until it seems that my husband is deliberately, perversely driving slowly. 'Go faster,' I groan as the traffic lights stay on red for much longer than they ever have before.

My husband's consideration for me is excruciating. 'We must stay calm,' he says. In the lobby of St John's Hospital, he pauses to buy me a Mars bar from a snack dispensing machine. 'In case you need energy during the labour.'

'Hurry, please hurry,' I pant.

We pass oncology. I wonder if my mother is sleeping. We turn into the labour ward corridor. The hospital is as fluorescent and overlit as Myer Grace Brothers; another kind of overpriced dying house. There in the corridor I vomit splashily, impolitely over the gleaming pale grey linoleum.

'Sorry about the mess,' I mutter to the midwife. My True Body has abandoned me. There's barely a minute between each contraction now. I feel like a weak swimmer in enormous seas, almost unable to surface enough to breathe.

They lift me on to a high birthing couch. They shine an enormous bright light between my legs. My pudenda is like a prize bloom on display, lit up, on a pedestal. It's a long way for a prize bloom to fall.

'It's too high and bright up here. Give me the floor.' They help me to a low vinyl bed.

The midwife is wearing goggles. She bends to speak into my ear. 'Listen, Isabelle. The bad news first. The baby is posterior.'

I can't remember what that means. It sounds dire. Will I survive my baby? Will my baby survive me?

'The good news now. You're ten centimetres dilated. You're ready to go. The fastest first stage I've seen in a prima.'

I've come back to my True Body, I want to explain. It's in my family. We are ciap cheng. We begin labour in food halls, wet markets and dying houses. We are efficient and immoderate in all things.

Louise the obstetrician enters. She pulls on a green gown, rubber gloves, plastic goggles. She is so far away with her instruments, her expertise. She is ground control and I am in orbit. Such weight, such lightness.

'We going to the moon, Louise? Have my Mars bar.' The desperation of the motherless mother-to-be, bribing and joking with the obstetrician who will deliver her, trying to bring her closer.

*Huh huh ppphhh* . . . There is no pause between contractions now. There is no time for gas, for drips, for chewing on ice or chocolate.

Just this panting, this urgent lifting towards the True Body.

The midwife puts her face down close to mine. 'Are you listening? Because your baby is posterior, you have to keep pushing *after* the contractions are finished.'

I do, but I have never been taught the correct breathing for this. *Hupphhh-hu pphhh*. I think of my mother, lying in oncology, eyes closed, breathing quietly: *hph, hph*.

I am suddenly unaccountably certain something is about to break. 'I have to stop,' I say. 'Help me.'

They take this as a loss of will on my part. 'You mustn't. You *can* keep going.'

I do, with an effort that is beyond my muscles and

membranes. There are no signs readable on my body that anything has broken.

There is a burning around my perineum as the baby's head comes at it wider and wider. The obstetrician swabs at my stretched membrane with a sponge doused in anaesthetic. In Singapore, the Malay midwife bathed Rose's perineum in the juice of lime and water. Her midwife forwent the danger money.

In St John of God's, the midwife puts a mirror at the foot of my bed as the obstetrician watches the baby's heartbeat on a screen. My nose is red with burst capillaries, with having to sustain the pushing far beyond the contractions. It's as if my nose is a barometer to the pressure my backside is under.

'Keep pushing. The head's through now.'

*Ph-ph-phhhhhhhhh*.

I am no longer sure of my statistics. 40–46–, with my vagina and hips blown off the graph. I come into my True Body again. So that, strangely, I hardly feel my baby slide out from that point on, even when her shoulders come, the widest part of her body passing through me.

'There. Nothing broken. No episiotomy needed. Not even a tear.'

The obstetrician has a pink bundle in her arms and a piece of placenta on her goggles. She gives my husband scissors to cut the bloodied blue and cream umbilical cord.

'It's like cutting through rubber,' he says as the midwife wraps our baby and places her on my chest.

Hidden in the bundle of blankets is a little bald head, a face wrinkled by amniotic fluid and my body's contractions. She has her chin down on her chest and her hands together under it, as if she is praying. Venerable little monk. With fierce eyes, like a warrior's. There's a smear of vernix like warpaint on her brow. It's been quite a fight.

It's early dawn outside, a nacreous oyster-shell grey. I would like to see my mother. They ring the ward to find she's still not out of her anaesthetised sleep.

Perhaps my mother takes the deepest breaths of her life. Perhaps she becomes aware that she is breathing alone.

Perhaps she calls: 'Help me . . . Help me . . .' Does anyone hear? Her voice is possibly too thin. Perhaps she relives her fight to breathe in the dying house in 1960. Perhaps she is dreaming of rescue by the dying-house proprietor, that flash of white and gold, that graceless angel.

In the labour ward of St John's Hospital, we are all sure it is over. We are clowns with our wide smiles, my red nose. Except that there is more pain inside me, a slow steady build this time. No one has taught me about this one. Someone asks me a question but I can't respond. I am in shock at this new agony. I clench against it.

My arms loosen around the baby.

'Something's broken,' I say before my baby, the room, my husband's worried face are lost to me.

Perhaps my mother fights her way through shock too, back in the Singapore dying house; and here in the oncology ward below me. Perhaps that's why the Malay midwife wrapped my mother's abdomen in coconut oil and bandages, to bring her back to her body. Perhaps that's why she is still sleeping on the floor below me, under the layers of anaesthetic and green hospital gown.

When I wake, my breasts are like two Eskies packed full and hard with milk. I hardly recognise myself in the mirror.

'What broke?' I ask my husband.

'Blood vessel in the birth canal,' he says. It sounds so

nautical. 'Haematoma. Your bottom is blue with bruising.'

I hobble down to post-natal physiotherapy classes. I
wheel the baby down with me in her Perspex crib, afraid to
let her out of my sight.

'These exercises will do you good,' exhorts the phy-
siotherapist. 'They will give you back your figures. Now.
Take three deep breaths. Inhale. Exhale. Inhale. Exhale.
And again. Feel your breath enter your body.'

My body? Where is my True Body?

Somewhere in the hospital below me, surely my mother
breathes, that sound like the beating of wings on air
searching for somewhere safe.

# Living Death: An Online Elegy
## *Hannah Fink*

I was wearing a pale blue seersucker hospital gown that joined at the nape of the neck with Velcro – I had taken my nightie off as it was soaked with blood and amniotic fluid – sitting on the very edge of the bed standing on the points of my toes, neither standing up nor sitting down, saying to the anaesthetist in a tiny voice, 'Help me.'

Then it was quiet. I had stopped vomiting and trembling, and the pain was gone. It was just Tessa and me and Andrew in the big pink room. Dr Grey had gone home. Tess said to Andrew, 'There's a little red button next to the bed. Push it if I tell you to.' And then, gently, slowly, he came. I could feel the contractions through the anaesthetic. It was the most perfect stillness. Tess turned his head around, and delivered his body. 'It's a beautiful little boy,' said Tessa. Andrew burst into inconsolable sobs. Tessa cleaned him, measured him, wrapped him, then brought him to me. I was so happy holding him – I was so happy to see him. He was exactly who I thought he was when I was carrying him. Tessa took some photos of us together and I look just as a mother does gazing with love at her infant.

We buried him at Rookwood the next day. Cantor Deutsch sang a brief prayer; Andrew wrapped his coat around the little coffin. It was painted tar black; I thought it would be pine like Papa's coffin. I put a photo of Andrew and me in the grave, smiling to the brim on our wedding day. We passed the shovel between us – me, Andrew, Dad, Mum, John, Ben, Aunty Bev, Phil, Sole, Anne, Aunty Jenny, Tessa. The gravedigger put a Letraset sign on top of the little mound: BABY SHAPIRO. He has a name but it is not spoken.

When we buried Papa two months earlier, the marker on his grave was handwritten in spiky capitals. JACK FINK, it read, and it was impossible to believe someone of such great will and wit could be contained in that small mound of earth. His death to me was as appalling, as outrageous as that of a young person. 'It's your grrrandtfader here,' Papa would say in his Bialystocker accent when he telephoned, and implicit in the magnitude of my love for him is my failure to capture him beyond the grave, to make his peasant brilliance live.

I spent the seven days of Shiva staying at Grandma's. I looked for something, a talisman, that would keep Papa with me. *Dancing Rebecca*, his favourite record? Grandma wouldn't part with it. A tie? A *siddur*? He was not a man of objects, of things. In the kitchen I found a shopping list next to the telephone, written in his beautiful, curlicued migrant's hand. *Cheese, Tamatos, Milk, Eggs, Apples, Salman*. Papa could speak five languages and he was a self-made millionaire, but he never quite mastered written English. Nothing is more dear to me than this piece of paper. I fancy that a tiny part of his spirit is caught in the flourish of the T.

It was the day Jason came to connect my modem that I found out my baby was dead.

I had been tired, dreadfully tired, all weekend. By the time Jason came, on Monday, I could barely stand up and I had lost my voice. I tried to sit beside him as he fiddled with my password – HANDBAG 1 – but had to lie down. I rang the doctor, and said, without even having thought it,

'I haven't felt the baby move today.' I had already rung once that day and been dealt the usual sedative platitudes fed pregnant women – *it's perfectly normal* – but the receptionist didn't say that, she said, 'Come in straight away.' So I went in to Jason, who was tip-tapping away on my keyboard, and said, 'I have to go out for a minute. There's something wrong with my baby.'

Sitting in the waiting room of the ultrasound clinic, I put my hand on my mother's arm and said, gently as one might to a child, 'You know that the baby might be dead.' I still don't know how I could have said that, because I hadn't thought it. My baby's dead. My baby died. I had a baby that died. The words were as unbelievable then as now.

I knew it could happen. My second cousin Naomi died of pre-eclampsia with her baby still in her womb. She was seven months' pregnant and she had had an ideal pregnancy until that day. I knew unnatural death, too. My first boyfriend, Blake, was killed in a car accident when he was just twenty-two. His preternatural beauty and brilliance lent a false logic to his death – we sang 'Vincent' by Don McLean at his funeral – but I learnt then, after two years of crying, that things didn't make sense.

It was when the radiologist said, 'Are you going back to see Dr Grey?' that the silence weighing on me buckled, and I knew.

I rang my friend Tessa and told her my baby was dead. Tessa is a midwife. I met her ten years ago in the Evening Star Hotel in Surrey Hills when I was in a band called Pressed Meat and the Smallgoods. I went to hospital the next day. Tessa came in an hour or so after I was admitted. I knew if I kept looking at her beautiful smiling face I would be OK. She showed me how to make the bed-head move. 'Bed goes up, bed goes down,' she said, quoting Homer Simpson. I thanked Tessa for coming in when she wasn't working. 'I would do anything for you, Hannah,' she said.

It wasn't until six weeks later that I actually went online, my first venture into the Net. I typed in STILLBORN, and was asked to provide a subsidiary term. STILLBORN + INFAMY, one of the offerings, got me ORDER FROM CHAOS: Stillbirth Machine/Chrushed Infamy. On www.hannah-h.org/loss.html I found Hannah's Prayer E-Mail Pal and Prayer Support Connection, which has its own quarterly publication, *Hannah to Hannah (H2H)*. STILLBORN + INTRAUTERINE revealed SANDS Australia, but the link didn't work.

Then I found my group. It is a board where mothers of stillborn babies write letters to one another. It was the first site I found and I've never gone anywhere else since.

Over the next year I spent countless hours weeping and laughing into the green glare of my computer screen as I read missives from Karen and Carrie and Shannon and Sharon, from Myrna, Nina, Rebekah, Cindy, Mindy, Jodi, Julie, Jan and Justina. I loved these women fiercely, wholly, and we poured the love we could not give our dead children on one another. We were all in the sorrowing no-man's-land between having had our babies and trying to conceive again, a nowhere in which time is measured by ovulatory cycles and trimesters, birth days and death days. So while we obsessively talked about temperature charting, mittelschmerz, and the quality of menstrual blood, we also talked about our babies, our husbands (there were no single or gay mothers) and our grief. Our intimacy was forged in words, tears and endless descriptions of cervical mucus.

Months went by before I realised that what I was doing was participating in a self-help group. And as a Net naif, everything would strike me as novel, ingenious. 'Just lurking,' a casual visitor would announce, and I would be struck by the wit of the phrase, little realising that this was everyday Net speak. Being slow-witted myself, the delays of letter-writing suited me better than live chat; it also promoted the kind of thoughtfulness necessary in a group where everyone was still sharp with pain.

Except for me, Padma from Singapore, Sarah from Warwick and Debbie from Darwin, all the women were American. I was at once charmed and nauseated by their Americanness. There was so much that was galling – calling each others 'ladies', for a start. 'Hey, ladies, how about a rollcall. I'll go first. ++++ vibes!!!!!!!!' The cheer-leading. The exclamation marks. The miles of bad poetry (which always contained the words 'angel', 'tears', 'Mom-my', 'heaven', 'Jesus', 'love' and 'rosebud'). Some women degenerated into writing wretched, rambling letters to their babies. Others posted memorial web pages, as though the Internet were heaven itself, index of God's mind.

My correspondents were simultaneously unabashed and puritan: mawkish, effusive, bubbly, *sincere*. Yet I admired their openness, their confidence, their sense of play. They shared a freewheeling cultural freemasonry of which they were unaware and in which I longed to participate. Being American was evidently great fun. And there was a generosity, a womanly good-humoured-ness. Soon any ambivalence I'd had was lost. More than anything I longed to be able to say 'YOU GO GIRL!'

It took me a while to learn the protocols of the group. There were rituals of welcome and condolence, cheer squads (GO SPERMIES GO!!), and even an eccentric system of acronyms for things to do with fertility (so AF stood, inexplicably, for Aunt Flo – a menstrual period – whose unwelcome visit would often be preceded by her dog Spot). The advent of a period was received with commiseration, and the announcement of a pregnancy with jubilance. There were set pieces: the birth (or, in the case of a Caesarean, operation), the funeral, the gravestone, the empty cot, on first seeing a living baby or hearing that a friend was pregnant, and the anniversaries of conception, birth and death. Together we trawled over the things that haunted and punished us: the test we forgot to take, the party we should have skipped, the work we should have refused.

When I discovered the site I didn't realise that it was new and still in the process of invention – I assumed everyone was an Internet habituée and knew the rules of the game – and so I delivered my first post with some trepidation:

My baby was delivered at 33 weeks on 29 October last year. He was my first child. He had died in utero some days before. I was put on drugs for two days to induce labour then the doctor broke my waters. Very swiftly I went into full labour. I was incredibly fortunate to have a very dear friend who is a midwife who delivered him.

His birth was beautiful (after the pain, when I was on the epidural, that is) – strangely, it was still the most wonderful thing, even though I knew he was dead – and he was a beautiful baby. He looked just like his father and half-sister.

I had a million tests done and the doctor said that the cause of death was foetal-maternal transfusion – that is, the baby haemorrhaged into my bloodstream through an imperceptible fault in the placenta. He had only heard of this once in his career fifteen years ago. They don't know how or why it happened. My pregnancy was a healthy one. There was nothing wrong with my baby or with me. Although the doctor has spoken to me twice about it I don't understand what actually happened.

I then went on with a lengthy catalogue of my every anxiety: about my menstrual cycles, my teeth falling out, my grandfather's death, my grandmother's grief, et cetera, et cetera, et cetera. Not the way to post, I realised, when I got only three responses, compared with Angie, who posted a single paragraph immediately after me and who got no less than eight replies. 'Thank you', it was titled:

> I can't thank you enough for having this site. I have spent the majority of my day here reading, re-reading, crying and laughing. I lost my son Tyler last Wednesday, at twenty weeks. All my feelings and thoughts were posted here as I read through your messages. It is truly a comfort to know that there are people who understand, and it helps to know that it will get better with time. How did people make it through those first weeks? I have another son who is two and a half and I am having trouble coping with him and this loss. Any suggestions?

At first I was terribly hurt that only three people had responded – I had cried so hard reading their stories – but then realised it was because I hadn't pitched my post right. In contrast, Angie's message had all the hallmarks of the perfect post: brevity, a direct emotional response, a clear question and, above all, immediacy. Immediacy is the marrow of electronic meaning; its effect is cumulative yet very much located in space and time. There is no point in printing posts, as by the time the ink is dry any meaning will have expired: like a shiny black river rock that glints underwater, once collected it loses its sheen.

For months I did it all wrong. I would read all the posts, then mull over which ones if any I would respond to. Then I would cut and paste the post into my word processor, compose my reply, then paste it back on to the bulletin board. Being part of a community network, I had only two hours a day online, and I needed to spend them carefully.

Yet when I'd finished writing down how I felt, and fiddling a little with it – fixing commas, changing the odd word, deleting things that might make me sound too brainy, too much like a writer – somehow I couldn't feel it any more. I'd read back what I'd written and it would seem false, ornate – writerish. The way I wrote and how I read was perverted by my relationship with words. Where words to me were magic tokens, beautiful ornaments, vessels of truth, to my correspondents they were things you use in order to speak.

Writing, I realised, was something I had to get over. I'd find myself extemporising into cul-de-sacs where I knew my meaning would be lost by my readers because there was none. Or at least any meaning that mattered. I learnt to write only when I had to, when I was desperate: the pleasure in writing was not in the writing itself but in knowing that I had said what I meant. Gradually, eventually, I lost the little person sitting in my brain who evaluated people according to their syntax or their spelling or vocabulary, the fear that prompts irony and distrust: finally, writing and reading became purely subjective – a language of love.

The grief of a mother may be inexpressible but it is also encyclopedic, and our project was the communal articulation of our experience. 'I feel like I am deaf and dumb,' said Myrna, and as we moved our hands over our keyboards we began, painstakingly, to decipher the unwritten world in which we had found ourselves. Writing was very much about the articulation of pain, as though in capturing it in words it would remain captive, be staunched, and from the mire of feeling, words became oracular, astonishing. Yet our writing was as much an articulation as a transubstantiation. The meaning of the percussive

242

AAARGHS, OOOOOS, GRRRRS and YAAAAYS that punctuated our letters was guttural, visceral: when we pressed 'Post your message' we sent little shots of pure emotion coursing through the electronic currents that linked us. There is perhaps no word more poignant, more replete, than *Oh* – more a sound or a breath, a sigh, than a word – and it is through these sounds, the invisible capillaries of chatter, that feeling travels.

We came to share one another's language, to speak a common tongue. Our letters were threaded one to the next, stitched together with a borrowed phrase, a common word, a caught sentiment. Reading my later posts I barely recognise myself: I lost the I of writing and could only write in the corporate voice that we had become. 'Sometimes when I read your posts I think you must be able to see inside my mind,' says Nina; or, 'Reading your response was like talking to myself,' a common refrain. Soon there was no I: we had become one person.

Well, almost. Insincerity, I discovered, is a vital component of female friendship, and the capacity of women for becoming one another – for empathy – often arrives at a loss of self. I developed irrational dislikes for certain members, and equally irrational fondness for others. I was astonished to find myself feeling pangs of envy – that Sharon did not reply as warmly to me as she did to Shannon, that everyone fussed over Jennifer as though she were a child, that Maureen all of a sudden stopped replying to my posts – and, worse, to find myself competing for the affections of the other women. As much as I wanted to be understood, I wanted to be liked, I wanted to be *popular*. I would stare aghast at the screen in these realisations, appalled by my petty schoolyard jealousy, my vanity. The screen may be a window but it is also a mirror.

I loved Karen best, and I loved her straight away. She always managed to say exactly the right thing, and her voice to me was one of pure reason and pure love. I wrote for Karen and read for her responses; I had made her my ideal correspondent. But I loved Karen as much for her perfect punctuation as for her kindness and wisdom: I had fallen in love with her literacy. Because our relationships were comprised entirely of words, I made the mistake of confusing articulateness with goodness, literacy with eloquence. It was often the less literate writers who were able to speak the most clearly. 'I am so depressed all the time I feel like a dead person inside a living body,' wrote Shannon, and I was riveted by the rightness of her phrase – it hit me with all the force of a cliché realised. I had written reams trying to articulate how I felt and there it all was in eight words.

Darlene has gone into premature labour on *Roseanne*. She is in hospital, and her baby is going to die. The whole episode is about the family, mainly the women, coming to terms with the fact of the baby's impending death. I sat with Andrew and Anna through its twenty-four minutes' crying, a continuous stream of water falling from my wide eyes, transfixed by the flickering colours in the little box, thankful, released. I couldn't believe what I was seeing and hearing. I was so grateful to *Roseanne* for representing us, at last. My heart was opened. This is what is meant by catharsis.

But then the baby lived. It was a miracle – a sitcom miracle. What bitter salt for my wound. 'Wouldn't it be good if shows didn't always have the right ending?' said Anna.

'But can I ask you,' said my psychiatrist in her Indian accent, 'who *is* Roseanne?'

I went to a shrink so she could tell me that what I felt was normal. I spent most of the time entertaining or shocking her with all the stupid things people say. Like

'Don't you want to know what's *really* wrong with you? I mean, the *psychological* reason you can't have children?' Or the standards: 'You weren't ready to have a child', 'Are you over it yet?' or, 'Have you thought of adopting?' 'Well, you know,' said Andrew's best friend, one, I was to learn, who was incapable of dealing with death, 'infant mortality was commonplace before this century.' Did women in the nineteenth century love their children less because they were more likely to die?

Losing a baby is very different from other kinds of deaths. It is a physical mourning, a bodily grief. One carries about oneself a constant, palpable absence, like wearing an empty knapsack. It is a diminishing experience. It makes you weak, depressive and slightly agoraphobic. And it is terribly lonely. You are ostracised from the world of pregnancy and of motherhood – pregnant women and new mothers are the first to shun you – and you fast learn that it is unwise to discuss your baby or your body with anyone. To do so is to invite them to say the wrong thing. What has happened to you is unimaginable, and so unwittingly people say the most grievous things.

'I'm convinced it's just ignorance,' says Mom09, writing to Shantele:

> I remember when I had no problem getting pregnant and carrying a baby to term. I just assumed that it was just as easy for everyone else. And I admit that I was guilty of saying some pretty ignorant things to people who had a problem pregnancy or couldn't get pregnant. If I had all of their numbers or addresses now, I would call each one of them and apologise for being so insensitive. So I will apologise to you, for them, to try to start making up for all of the times that I was ignorant.

I was so shocked the first time I walked down a street not pregnant and someone bumped into me. Pregnant women are hallowed beings for whom crowds part, cars stop, strangers smile. But just as a pregnant woman is a sacred object, so a mother of a dead child becomes an object of fear, a pariah. She is the embodiment of every pregnant woman's worst phantasms; she is a living death.

Last summer Tessa and I often met to go swimming at the Icebergs. We sat in the sun chatting and looking at all the different shapes of women – the stubby middle-aged Russians, the rake-thin teenagers, the jelly-thighed new mothers – and among everything else we talked about, Tess would tell me about the deliveries she'd done that week and I would tell her about what was happening with the women in my group.

One noon as we were sitting looking out to sea I felt two small hands on my shoulders and heard a little boy say, beseechingly, *Mummy*. He had mistaken me for his mother, who also had short dark hair and a black swimming costume. I could feel his wet lips on my ear, and I didn't so much hear as feel the absolute trust and intimacy of his small voice, deep in my body as though from inside a sea shell. For one second I knew what it felt like to be the mother of a living child, to live in the world of motherhood.

RE: THE LATE SHAPIRO; BABY who passed away on Wed 29/10/1997 (29th Tishri 5758).

To erect a single memorial stone as follows:

Grey granolite [cement composite mixture] headstone/ desk lying flat on the ground and inclined at the back with a FLUSH BELFAST black South African granite panel 14″ × 22″ × 1″ polished face only, edges sawn [unpolished] finish. Including ALL the raised-polished, natural, everlasting letters, the sum of . . . $690.00

There is a line to be crossed and at a certain point the highly unnatural activity of spending all day writing to people you've never met becomes ordinary. But after spending four or five hours thinking and writing to all the day's correspondents, realising that the day had in fact gone, and that I was quite spent for it, the evanescence of my friends, of our link, would strike me, and I would fend off the thought that our bond was as fragile as the lives of our children, and as random as their deaths. I knew it couldn't last, that our friendships were ephemeral and, quite literally, insubstantial. That which bound us would pass, and we would be drawn back into the cycle of life, some of us with children, some without.

I rarely post nowadays. I don't know anyone in the group any more, as almost all my friends have moved on. Last month Kate gave birth to Krystal Rose, LeeAnn to Trevor and Angie to Tanner Christian. Karen and Carrie are pregnant, Karen courtesy of IVF, Carrie of Clomid. Shannon has disappeared. I lurk occasionally, but the tone is not so thoughtful, the women seem more cavalier. It took hundreds of thousands of words to get to know my friends, and I don't seem to have the heart to invest in the new crowd. Disconcertingly, a couple of months ago the site hub crashed, and all our archives are now irretrievable.

On the anniversary of my baby's death I went with Tessa to Rookwood. It is such a long drive there that arriving always comes as a small shock. A dog had shat on his grave. I didn't mind; at least it was compostible. The grave is near the kerb of a road and the earth in which he is buried is unnatural, full of asphalt and bitumen. Tess had brought some white roses, which she placed over the dog shit.

The day before, Tessa had asked if I wanted her to come with me to the cemetery and I had dallied, not wanting to prevail on her kindness. But then I realised that she wanted to go – he was her baby, too.

The only answer to radical loss, said Rabbi Fox at our baby's consecration, is radical love. And there I think of Tess. I stop, stilled by the thought of her great grace and beauty – I can still feel her gentle midwife's hands pressing my abdomen, still see her dear face as she brought my son from me. Out of love, from friendship, Tessa made the worst day of my life the most miraculous thing.

There is a grease-stained fingerprint on the top right-hand corner of page 199 of my *Urtext Mozart Sonatas*. It is Blake's fingerprint: he had turned the page for me while I was playing and he was eating fish and chips. I think of him sitting beside me every time I play Köchel 333, and I remember how I snapped at him for blemishing the page.

Blake is dead now – he has been dead for fifteen years – and apart from that fingerprint I have an old pyjama top and a gingham shirt he loved. They have not smelled of him for years. I have a few photographs. But I also have a small suitcase of his letters, letters to me. His mother burnt my letters to him, thinking that I didn't want them, that she would preserve our intimacy by destroying them. He died all over again the day she told me she had burnt my letters: it was the end of our conversation.

My baby did write to me, a long black line down the middle of my torso. It has faded now, my linea nigra, been rubbed off; there are crumbly remnants in my belly button. How proud I was of this tattoo – it was his message to me, his love letter. My memorial, my love poem to my dear little baby, is thousands of words floating in cyberspace, everlasting words inaccessible in links that are now lost.

# Life with Danny

## *Nick Hornby*

It wasn't Danny's mental development that concerned us at first. For a start, there were too many other things to worry about: he was born by emergency Caesarean after a complicated labour, during which his mother, Virginia, became dangerously ill, and very soon afterwards he required an operation for an inguinal hernia, and he was slow to crawl and even slower to walk. But these problems seemed to be righting themselves, and reasonably thorough neurological investigations revealed nothing untoward, and in any case he had begun to acquire language. He babbled and then said 'ball' and when he handed us something he said 'Eye'ar' in his much-loved childminder's Glaswegian accent, and for a few weeks, at the beginning of 1995, when he was fifteen months old, we almost began to relax.

In the spring of that year, however, he crashed, in the way that computers crash. He went haywire. The acquisition of language stopped; worse than that, he lost nearly all the words he had been using regularly. He would become catatonic if we went out anywhere, especially to places where there were other children – he would demand to be picked up, and then slump over a parental shoulder, avoiding eye-contact with anybody. For a time we tried to convince ourselves that this was an extreme reaction to the departure of the Glaswegian childminder and her little girl, and that he would shake himself out of his obliviousness to the world at any moment.

I can remember waking up morning after morning, thinking, Today's the day he'll say something, or show an interest in one of his toys, and at the time the hope was just as debilitating as any as yet undiagnosed disability, because we ended each day frantic with concern. We had friends with children born at the same time – on the same day, even – and these children were pulling away from Danny week by week; they were getting older, becoming toddlers, speaking in sentences, whereas Danny was actually regressing. It was as though we were watching what we had imagined to be 'normal' parenthood disappearing over the horizon.

Paradoxically he wasn't, and had never been, particularly difficult to look after. He wasn't curious, and so showed no desire to stick scissors into electrical sockets, or eat dog faeces, or climb up drainpipes on to sloping roofs; he liked nothing better than to sit in his bedroom on his own, looking at picture books and listening to music.

For a time, in fact, it was rather like sharing a house with a very small teenager, but his ability to amuse himself was no consolation because it indicated that this child was not like other children.

In the summer of 1995 a paediatrician told us, in a curiously offhand way, that Danny was handicapped, although nobody was sure precisely what form this handicap took (it was to be another year before he was finally diagnosed as autistic) and the vagueness was frightening.

He was still, or so it seemed to us, regressing; he was hardly using any words at all now, and he had begun to get fits of the giggles at inappropriate moments. He had always rocked backwards and forwards and flapped his arms, but now these habits had begun to look positively sinister, and his obsessive interest in doing the same puzzles over and over again was just as alarming. It was, for a while, possible to imagine everything and anything.

Maybe Danny's language would come back, and he would stop the rocking and giggling. Maybe he would disappear altogether. (In the awful days straight after the initial diagnosis it became possible to spiral further and further downwards, into a black pit where he had some terrible disease that would kill him sooner rather than later.)

What made things worse was that we could be told, by friends or professionals, at any stage of any day, whatever we wanted to hear. Well-meaning friends and relatives assured us that there was absolutely nothing wrong with Danny, and that professionals were scaremongers who were only interested in covering their backs; it was also clear that if we looked hard enough, we could find some specialist somewhere who could put our minds at rest.

We did see a couple of people like that, and for a few hours afterwards we felt relieved, elated even . . . but meanwhile, Danny was sitting in a corner somewhere, rocking and playing with his jigsaws, oblivious to most things, but especially to comforting diagnoses. A lot of the reassurance offered to us was predicated on there being nothing wrong with Danny at all, and once our fears had been confirmed, there was nothing much left for these people to say, beyond vaguely embarrassed murmurs of sympathy.

Meanwhile, Danny continued developing in his own erratic way. He had jettisoned almost all language, beyond five key words: the names of his four favourite television characters, and 'duddle' (i.e. cuddle) which could mean anything from 'I want to go to bed' to 'I have now finished my supper'.

That, he seemed to have decided, would do him, as far

as language went, and you could sort of see his point. He knew he would be fed and watered, he could kip when he felt like it, and 'duddle' ensured that he would be transported from one activity to the next. He had all the bases covered, all needs catered for – apart from the need for Postman Pat ('Bobat') and Fireman Sam ('Ma'), a need which he clearly felt was worth maintaining a language to express.

Otherwise, he 'borrowed' words for a short period of time, and then returned them to the shelf. 'Dog' came and went, as did 'Grandma' and even 'yeah': for a long time, well over a year, we could communicate with him by asking him a (very basic) question, usually connected with crisps or swings, which he would either answer in the affirmative or ignore completely – a useful, occasionally crucial, tool.

One morning, however, he woke up and decided that 'yeah' had outlived its usefulness, and we have never heard it again since in its proper context. It is impossible sometimes not to regard this kind of withdrawal as wilfully perverse.

The diagnosis of autism, when it eventually came, was hardly a surprise. By then we had learned enough, from books and from professionals and other parents, to know that much of Danny's developmental pattern and behaviour belonged on the autistic continuum, to use one of the many phrases with which we have become depressingly familiar over the last couple of years. (Some autistic kids attend mainstream schools; others don't even recognise their own parents. We are lucky in that Danny knows us and is demonstrative in his affection for us.)

Autism is a developmental neurological disorder that affects more than one in five hundred children; typically, the autistic child does not gesture, or make eye-contact, or speak, gets locked into inappropriate routines and behaviours, and cannot play imaginatively. In most cases the cause of the disorder is unknown, although there is a recognised genetic and organic component. Very occasionally the autistic child has a special pocket of talent, but parents of autistic children can get very fed up with repeatedly being told that their child will end up as a concert pianist or a great artist – there are a couple of television documentaries and films that have a lot to answer for. Basically, autism is very bad news.

Being given a label was helpful, up to a point, because we could begin to plan Danny's future in a way that ignorance had prevented us from doing properly hitherto. The choices, however, were bewildering. We could take Danny to the Higashi school in Boston, where his autism would be assaulted at all hours of the day and night. He could undergo psychotherapy (although it was hard to see quite how this would work, given that he was only able to use words that pertained to animated firemen and postmen). We could change his diet, we could swing him upside down, we could play him music backwards, there was this programme and that programme . . . if someone had suggested that we stick his head in a bucket containing iced water and a cauliflower twice a day, we would have listened with weary interest and headed off to the greengrocer's.

And there was no one to tell us which of these treatments were barmy, and which might trigger something in Danny: nobody in the NHS has the time or the information or, of course, the money to be able to sift through it all.

It is easy to become evangelical about treatments which you believe have helped your child. This evangelism comes from the best possible place inside you – a desire to help others whom you know for a fact, because you have been there, to be frightened and confused and desperate. I understood this when others were telling us to ring this person and that organisation; it was just that there were so many pieces of conflicting advice that for a while we felt paralysed. Eventually we were put in touch with a couple of people we trusted simply because their conviction was so strong that we could not help but listen and believe, and in any case, the treatment they recommended, a home-based behavioural therapy pioneered in (of course) the United States by Professor Ivor Lovaas, made perfect sense.

Danny is now six months into the programme and making progress, and as a consequence, Danny's mother and I are as evangelical as the parents who introduced us to the method in the first place. We are currently involved in trying to set up TreeHouse, a school for autistic children in north London, where behavioural therapy will form the basis of the teaching.

Behavioural methods such as Lovaas break developmental steps down into tiny pieces, and the child is made to do things over and over again until he (and the pronoun is appropriate, because the autistic child is usually a he) has mastered them. This is not as robotic as it sounds – Danny loves his therapy (and his therapists). For a start, it makes him feel successful, and he is motivated to learn. And anyway, his efforts are rewarded by the things he loves – rough and tumble play, sweets, anything that keeps him going. What is remarkable about Lovaas and similar methods is that its specialists – not quacks, but qualified university professors – talk quite routinely about 'recovering' children. Believe me, such talk awakens one's interest.

Autistic children do not copy, because they are oblivious to much of the outside world, and because they do not copy, they do not learn; Danny's therapists have taught him to copy, by making him focus and prompting him and rewarding him and praising him. He will now attempt to copy simple words, and if you tell him to say 'hello' he will do so. If you are the parent of a child who has developed normally, this will sound heartbreakingly inadequate; if you are the parent of an autistic child who has never heard your son's voice properly, you will know what an enormous and enthralling breakthrough this is.

Autistic children do not play with many toys, because they do not understand the value of trains and cars and dolls and other representational toys, but Danny's therapists are teaching him what to do.

Some of it works and some of it doesn't, and there is a lot of trial and error, and everything takes for ever, and it is frighteningly expensive – Danny has thirty-three hours of therapy a week, and someone flies from America every three months to monitor his progress – but there is research to indicate a success rate of 47 per cent with pre-school autistic children, if Lovaas's methods are rigorously applied. From where we have been standing, that looks an impossibly rich, fat, high number.

Danny's treatment has given his parents two things: hope, because he has made more progress in the last six months than he had made in the previous couple of years, and a sense of relief born from the knowledge that we are doing the best we can for our son at the moment. But none of it is easy, and Danny will always be autistic.

He still cannot speak, he is still nowhere near being toilet-trained, his sleep is poor, and neither of us knows what the future holds. Just recently the NHS started to deliver his nappies, which is our entitlement as the parents of a disabled child, and as I was putting one on the other day, I noticed that his size had changed from large to small, and it was hard to ignore the symbolism here. The label was telling me that he was no longer a toddler finishing off a stage of his development. He was now a young disabled person, and the disability was here to stay; the nappies will only get bigger and bigger.

It's at moments like that you need all the hope you can find.

*Donations to the TreeHouse Trust can be sent c/o AMP Ltd, 396 St John's Street, London EC1V 4NJ. For information about the Lovaas method, and donations, contact PEACH, PO Box 10836, London SW13 9ZN.*

# In the Stars

## *Rosie Waitt*

I'm sitting next to Tim in the van, daydreaming, hands cradling my rounded belly, the baby lulled quiet by the engine and the gentle rhythm of the road. In the back, the children are asleep, mouths wide open, red hot faces and damp sticking hair. When they wake we will stop for lunch and after lunch we will move on again. We're not going anywhere in particular, just meandering, letting one thing lead to the next.

After months on the road our days have formed a regular rhythm. Sometimes the children cry and grumble and the van fills with a sharp tension. Sometimes they play happily together and Tim and I spend time savouring long conversations. Often we sing along to children's tapes, songs and nursery rhymes, played over and over. But there are also quiet times like now, when the children sleep or just stare out. Then we pass hours moving through flat landscape with low bush, termite mounds for as far as we can see, dry riverbeds, the occasional car . . . Regularly we see kangaroos, usually dead on the side of the road, their bodies swollen with the heat, or carcasses half devoured by wedge-tailed eagles who rise into the sky as we pass. The monotony has its own sort of beauty. There's something hypnotic about it, something about the vast expanses that makes us look inward.

And backwards, back to the sticky heat of outback Northern Queensland. Six, seven months ago when the line unexpectedly turned blue on the thin strip of litmus paper I was holding. We were staying with Greg and Kerry Jonnson at their organic cattle station. It was hot there, hot and sticky, clouds building up and up, and time slowing down, as we waited for the wet season to begin.

'You're pregnant,' Tim had said the previous night, certain he could read the signs.

'Don't be silly,' I replied. But the next day I was less certain. One of Greg and Kerry's daughters, Michelle, wandered over looking terribly ill. She sat with me for a few minutes.

'God, I feel awful,' she said. 'I must be pregnant.'

Then later, Tina (a daughter-in-law) mentioned that she too might be pregnant.

'Me too,' I said without thinking.

Within minutes Shane (the eldest son) showed up and looked me over. 'You pregnant?' he asked.

'I don't know,' I said, nervous now and feeling uncomfortably like one of his cows.

'I'm driving into Townsville tomorrow to pick up tests for the others,' he said. 'I'll get you one too.'

I nodded, aware that underneath my embarrassment was a strong sense of relief. It was out of my hands.

The next afternoon the children slept, naked, with arms flung everywhere in the heat. I opened all the windows to let in any stray breeze, but there was nothing, hardly enough oxygen to keep breathing. The atmosphere was getting heavier, even more humid, and so still I could feel the tension in the air. My head was throbbing, filled with pre-storm positive ions. It was almost certainly going to rain. But when?

'The dust is coming,' shouted Kerry, her words breaking through the heavy silence and startling me into motion. In the homestead doors and windows were slamming shut, one resounding bang after another. Looking out, I could see a disturbance of some kind on the horizon, a red cloud coming this way, fast. I raced to close the windows and zip up the door, not quite making it before a huge roar and an immense gust of wind stopped me in my tracks. The tent heaved to one side and then righted itself, but the children didn't stir. I still had to close the windows and that meant going out there again. For just a few seconds dust swirled in the atmosphere, stinging me with its ferocity. Then came the rain, big heavy drops, plopping, almost sizzling, on the hot earth. Steam rose from the ground, a glorious smell, like the freshly ironed clothes I wore as a child. There was no time to savour it because the wind was fast becoming ferocious, pushing the tent one way and then the other. Back inside there were already puddles on the floor and the table and chairs had been knocked over by the heaving canvas. But the children slept on. I slid their bunks away from the sides of the tent and prepared to sit it out. Moments later the first pole broke and I knew we'd have to move. So I unzipped the front, letting the wind fill the tent like a balloon. God, I thought, imagining us flying across the outback, now it's about to take off. Quickly, and with a strength that only comes with emergencies, I tucked one sleepy child under each arm and ran over to the homestead, thinking as I went, that if I was pregnant I really shouldn't be doing this.

The temperature had dropped fifteen degrees in a few minutes, and I left Nikita and Freda wet and shivering in the house, while I went back to get clothes and towels and secure the tent. The storm exhausted itself quickly, turning into a slow drizzle and then drying up altogether. I was a nervous wreck. 'Stop,' I wanted to shout, 'I've had en-ough!' but after a five-year drought the Jonnson family were ecstatic and wanted to play, like kids in the mud. Everyone piled into four-wheel-drives and set out to in-spect the property, driving much too fast, sliding all over the road, ploughing through dips and over bumps. I sat in the back seat, with Nikita on my lap, a fixed smile on my face and the horrible wet taste in my mouth that meant I was going to be sick at any moment. Once again the thought popped into my head that if I was pregnant this wasn't a very good idea.

Back at the tent, we mopped up and waited nervously for Shane to return from his 700-kilometre round trip and distribute the pregnancy tests. It was just getting dark when I finally slunk off to the toilets, clutching my conspicuous packet. Not willing to share this moment, I stood in the cubicle waiting for the line to turn blue and when it did all I felt was the heavy weight of certainty settling inside me. Back outside, I was red-faced and shell-shocked, but there was no escaping the others. We were all positive. Three women on a remote cattle station. I laughed along with the 'something in the water' jokes but deep down I was worried. The timing really was appalling. We were only two months into a twelve-month trip. Was it safe to carry on, with the intense heat and rough roads and all the physical strains that camping entailed? Could I do it? I was already experiencing the debilitating lethargy of early pregnancy. Would it persist? How could Tim and I juggle work and the children? What about my writing? I knew from experience how scatty I get when I'm pregnant. How could I write and travel and be pregnant and be a good mother? And if I could do all that, could I do any of it well?

'We should have been more careful,' said Tim.

'Now what are we going to do?' I asked.

He shook his head. 'How did it happen?'

'Oh come on, you know exactly how it happened . . . and when.'

'It was that bottle of wine, wasn't it.'

I laughed. Working out the dates pulled everything back

into perspective for us. We realised this baby was conceived six weeks ago, at Undara – a very special place at a very special time.

'What a wonderful thing,' Tim said, and suddenly I understood what a gift we'd received. Our baby had chosen us, it had chosen its time and it was very welcome. We agreed to carry on. It might not be the practical thing, but it felt right.

And now, so many months later, it still feels right, I think, scanning the horizon for a tree, just a little shade to shelter us while we eat our lunch. There are no trees. By mid-afternoon hunger forces us to the side of the road. The temperature outside is in the high thirties and in just a few minutes the temperature inside rises to the mid-forties. Tim starts the engine again and leaves the air conditioning running. We sit huddled inside, eating our droopy sandwiches and drinking lukewarm water, surrounded by a vast dazzling heat which makes the air wobble into luscious mirages.

'I need the toilet, Mummy.'

Stepping out into the sunlight I stretch painfully, relieved to feel the heavy ache in my womb lighten a little. I inhale and gasp as hot air burns all the way down. Holding Nikita so she doesn't wee on her clothes, I watch the liquid darken the ground, sending steam and dust rising, before disappearing altogether only a few seconds later. The ground is littered with bones, bleached white by the sun and glistening. Bones. A landscape of death. It seems to me that this is a world entirely without sentiment, a place where death is inconsequential. I shudder and walk a bit further from the car, my hand moving involuntarily to the new life forming inside me. Standing in this impossible heat I feel the baby move. Now that I am uncurled, it is playful, free to kick and toss inside the sheltered wetness of my womb. Just a few thin layers between out here and in there.

I'm relieved to be back in the van, it feels safer in here, another wall to hold things at bay. Tim tells me that it is my turn to drive, but I feel dreamy and distant, a long way from this narrow straight highway. I am becoming vague about things, but this time I know that eventually my thoughts will sharpen again and I don't feel the need to battle for lucidity. I look down at my belly wedged in tight behind the steering wheel. There's a little girl inside, almost ready to join us. And for a moment the imminence of it all makes me panic because we don't have a name, nothing, except Harry and we can't call her that. I think about the ultrasound, how I lay back on a bed as a nurse rubbed gel into the cold metal instrument that would trace my baby's movements. We were all there, Tim and Nikita and Freda, watching our baby on a television screen, seeing its tiny little fingers curl and uncurl. I expected to feel something, but there was only irritation because my bladder was full and the nurse dismissive and I was suddenly repelled by all this cold clinical science around me.

'It's another girlie,' said the nurse, and I detected a note of triumph in her voice as she wiped at my greasy belly with a tissue. She turned away then, already moving on to the next patient, unaware of how casually she had taken the magic from us.

'She's spoilt it,' I said to Tim, wiping tears from my eyes. 'I didn't want to know.'

'Three girls,' said Tim, shaking his head. 'I'll be way outnumbered.'

We left the hospital, clutching a few blurry photographs of our new baby and the sure knowledge that we were having a girl.

A girl, I think, glancing back at Nikita and Freda, busy tearing an entire box of tissues into spaghetti strips for dinner. I like girls. Looking ahead again I see something and slam on the brakes, slowing just in time to watch an immense goanna plod across the road, oblivious to us and to its narrow escape from death. Just as I am beginning to relax again a road train approaches and I tense up, grasping the wheel harder, pulling slightly off the road to avoid the awful vacuum it creates as it passes. Unexpectedly, something hits the windscreen and fine cracks spread from the point of impact. I duck as another stone hits the glass.

'Jesus, what was that?' asks Tim, waking up with a start.

'A stone,' I say. 'Lucky it didn't break . . . I really don't fancy driving without . . . Oh God!' We have lost all visibility as the car plunges through a plague of locusts. Within seconds the windscreen is splattered with the insects, the wipers ineffective against this onslaught. Then just as suddenly they are gone. By this time, my knees have turned to jelly.

'OK,' I say, 'your turn. I've had enough.' I pull up by the side of the road and feel the wheels spin in the dirt. We're bogged. The baby tosses and turns, reacting to the fear that surges through us both. I feel very vulnerable and want to cry because the baby could come at any time and we are a long way from anywhere and I don't want her to be born out here. I don't want to squat in this dust, surrounded by locusts and bones and the stench of death. I don't want to watch my waters break and flood around me and evaporate in seconds. For the first time I'm afraid. I don't want to die. I don't want my baby to die.

As Tim digs us out of the dirt I stand watching, unable to help. I'm big and helpless and frustrated and I'm remembering all the advice we've had.

'Stop,' people said.

'Rent a house, have the baby, then decide what to do.'

'You're mad.'

'It's dangerous.'

'Think about the baby.'

Back then I felt strong enough to shrug off the weight of other people's opinions. Now, stranded on the side of an empty road, brushing flies out of the children's faces, wondering just how much water is left . . . now I am not so sure. Maybe they were right after all.

'Yay!' shout Nikita and Freda when Tim finally pulls the van on to the road. We are ready to set off again, but my hands are still trembling as I strap the children back into their seats and then haul myself up into the front. And by evening my sense of panic still hasn't subsided. We are living inside this little metal box in the middle of nowhere and the whole thing seems absurd. What are we doing here? The atmosphere is awful. It's still hot, but we have the windows shut because there are mosquitoes and I'm trying to do the dishes, but my belly is too big and every time I move in this tiny space it knocks something over. Up top the children are fighting and Freda screams in a way that pierces my eardrums. Tim tries to get past me, looking for pyjamas and toothpaste, but there's no way, so I have to climb outside to let him through. I can feel a hard heavy rage rising inside me and soon I know that something's going to give. But finally the clatter of the dishes is over and the children are asleep. A deep ringing silence fills the space around us and I can breathe again.

Later I brave the mosquitoes and stand outside, letting the cool and the dark embrace me, feeling my unspent rage subside. Looking up, all I can see is the vast expanse of stars, the rich, thick Milky Way smeared across the evening sky. I wonder about the stars, if this baby is written up there somewhere, in a language I can't read.

In the van I lie on my back, pressed down by the weight of the baby. There are stars inside too. It was in Undara that we made our own map of the sky, sticking a fluorescent galaxy on the ceiling of our van, so that the stars would accompany us everywhere. Undara National Park in the Gulf country of Northern Queensland. A park filled with massive volcanic tubes, formed 190,000 years ago. We nearly missed it. What then, I wonder? What would have happened to our baby? But at the last minute we turned and followed the signs and I was suddenly overcome with a sense of having arrived, not home, but somewhere we were meant to be. I remember the feel of the stone, the 300-million-year-old pink granite, how special it seemed. Good, or maybe just benign. Somehow wise. And the incredible tunnels, pitch black and cool, etched with extraordinary patterns by the flowing lava. And overriding all of these things was the sense of rightness at being in this place. Then, while the children slept above and the rain pelted around us, our baby was conceived. And now, thousands of kilometres later, in the far south-west corner of Australia, we are soon to meet.

In Albany everything is suddenly wet. It is raining. The rivers flow fast and wild and there is grass; green and soft. We find the house within an hour of arriving. It is one of those meant-to-be things. After nine months camping rough, this space is an extraordinary luxury. There are things we had stopped taking for granted. It is strange to have running water, a bath, a comfortable chair, a bed that is long enough, a fridge – things that give life a soft padding. Television is strange too, bright and intrusive, a white noise filling up the echoey silences of this house. Tim and I walk around tentatively, as if we have forgotten how to stretch our limbs. But Nikita and Freda have no qualms. Whooping with joy they race around and around, laying claim to their new space. The rain outside is not important any more. We are dry and there's room to move.

Now there is time for leisure. I sit at the kitchen table watching the southern right whales, resting or playing just off the shore. Or I take the children the short walk to the playground or the beach where they build sandcastles while I daydream. I eat voraciously and the babygrows, stretching my belly bigger and tighter. My mother arrives with her suitcase full of presents. She sits with me at the kitchen table, knitting booties for the baby. They're blue and I'm irritated.

'Mum,' I say. 'It's a girl.'

Soon I feel the restlessness and the need to walk and know that the baby is on its way. In the morning I walk around the coast, a slow painful waddle, punctuated with rest stops. I see seals basking on the rocks, dolphins playing amongst the breakers and immense whales sitting further out. That evening my waters break. I shower and dress, timing the contractions. Already they are strong. We haven't got long, I tell Tim. I kiss my sleeping children and shut the door behind me. Tomorrow everything will be different.

The labour is short, the contractions intense, but still I have a sense that everything is in slow motion. First there is the head, black hair, wet and matted, a purple face because the cord is wrapped tightly around its neck. Then there are tiny pink shoulders and in one great heave our baby emerges.

'It's a BOY!' I scream this out loud, so that the words fill the room, escape, travel down the corridor into other rooms and everyone knows. Tim looks up startled, eyes searching for what I have already seen. I am suddenly greedy.

'Give him to me, give him to me.'

I forget everything, the contractions, the stitches, everything. I just want to hold my baby tight. My little baby Harry. I look at Tim, at the tears streaming down his face and his smile. I cry at how happy he is. I am laughing and crying.

'He was supposed to be a girl,' I tell anyone who might be listening.

I look at him, his little face squeezed up against the light. He stretches his arms out, surprised at the absence of walls, and I see the alarm on his face at this frightening new freedom. Then I wrap him up tightly again and offer him my breast, watch his instincts at work as his mouth closes over my nipple. A boy. Conceived amongst the lava tubes and ancient pink granite of Undara. Formed on the road, to the rhythm of the engine and long slow days and dry dusty heat. And born in wet, cool Albany while the whales dance and sing in the ocean and rainbows hang in the sky. A boy.

And now we are five, I think, holding our little Harry tight. I feel a strong sense of completeness. Soon we will pack up and squeeze everything back into the van. Then we will set off again, up the west coast of Australia, into a landscape softened by spring. Through vistas of flowers growing from the deep red soil of the Pilbarra region. Daring colour combinations, reds and pinks, so many shades of purple, yellows, white . . . the wind blurring the colours. To exotic Broome where we will see Chinese dragons and Thai dancing and eat Japanese noodles, and to Darwin in 'troppo' season, with its impossible heat and colourful markets. And finally to the very heart of Australia and Uluru with its breathtaking serenity and strong presence, that no photograph could ever capture.

And then, a new home . . . somewhere. We will let it find us.

# ACKNOWLEDGEMENTS

I would like to acknowledge the generous assistance of the Royal Literary Fund, which has helped a number of the writers in this anthology, myself included.

*Jill Dawson*

*A Letter To Our Son* by Peter Carey. © Peter Carey, 1988. Reproduced by permission of the author c/o Rogers, Coleridge and White Ltd, 20 Powis Mews, London W11 1JN and first published in *Granta 24*, Summer, 1988 (Cambridge, UK)

*Deliverance* by Judith Bryan. © Judith Bryan, 2001

Extract from *East of the Mountains* by David Guterson. © David Guterson, 1999. Published by Bloomsbury (London, UK)

Extract from *The Snapper* by Roddy Doyle (Secker & Warburg), used by permission of The Random House Group Ltd (London, UK)

*Gwendolyn* by Alice Jerome. © Alice Jerome, 2001

*In the Stars* by Rosie Waitt. © Rosie Waitt, 2001. First published in *The Age*, 2002 (Melbourne, Australia)

*Taipei, Expectant* by Bernard Cohen. © Bernard Cohen, 2001. First published in *The Age*, 2001 (Melbourne, Australia)

# BIOGRAPHIES

Judith Bryan grew up in London with Jamaican and Guyanan heritage. Her first novel, *Bernard and the Cloth Monkey*, was published by Flamingo in 1998, and she is currently working on her second. She lives in London and has one son.

Peter Carey was born in Bacchus Marsh, Victoria, in 1943. He is the author of seven novels, *Bliss*, *Illywhacker*, *Oscar and Lucinda*, *The Tax Inspector*, *The Unusual Life of Tristan Smith*, *Jack Maggs* and *The True History of the Kelly Gang*; two short-story collections, *War Crimes* and *Collected Stories*; and *The Big Bazoohley*, for children. He has twice won the Booker Prize; for *Oscar and Lucinda* and *The True History of the Kelly Gang*. He lives in New York with his wife and two sons.

Bernard Cohen is an Australian writer, the author of four books – *Tourism*, *The Blindman's Hat*, *Snowdome* and *Hardly Beach Weather* – and of the CD-ROM *Foreign Logics* (with artist David Bickerstaff). *The Blindman's Hat* won the 1996 Australian/Vogel Literary Award. He was named three times on the *Sydney Morning Herald*'s Best Young Australian Novelists list and received a 2001 Arts Council of England Writer's Award. He currently lives in London with his partner and their two children.

Christopher Cyrill was born in 1970 and published his first novel *The Ganges and Its Tributaries* in 1993. His second novel *Hymns for the Drowning* was published by

Allen & Unwin in 1999. He is currently completing a hybrid book of essays and stories and steadily working on his third novel. He lives in Sydney and teaches fiction at Macquarie University.

Margo Daly is a travel writer and freelance editor and has published several short stories. She is the co-editor, with Jill Dawson, of *Wild Ways: New Stories about Women on the Road* (Sceptre UK, 1998). She was born in Sydney, where she now lives with her daughter.

Julia Darling lives in Newcastle-upon-Tyne in the north of England, and writes stories, novels and plays. She first started publishing stories in 1995, when her collection *Bloodlines* appeared. Many of her stories have been broadcast on national radio. Her first novel *Crocodile Soup* was longlisted for the Orange Prize. She is currently playwright in residence at Live Theatre in Newcastle, and is also an associate 'fellow' at Newcastle University, a post funded by the Royal Literary Fund.

Jill Dawson was born in England and is the author of three novels (all published by Sceptre): *Trick of the Light*, *Magpie* and *Fred & Edie*, which was shortlisted for the Whitbread Novel of the Year and the Orange Prize and longlisted for the IMPAC Award. She is also the editor of several anthologies, including with Margo Daly *Wild Ways* (Sceptre). She currently lives in the Fens, Cambridgeshire, with her partner and two sons.

Roddy Doyle was born in Dublin in 1958. His first novel *The Commitments* was published to great acclaim in 1987 and was made into a successful film by Alan Parker. *The Snapper* was published in 1990 and has also been made into a film, directed by Stephen Frears, as was his novel *The Van* (1991). *Paddy Clarke Ha Ha Ha* won the Booker Prize in 1993. His latest novel is *A Star Called Henry*.

Hannah Fink lives in Sydney, Australia. She is a former editor of *Art and Australia* and *Art AsiaPacific* magazines. She writes mostly about art and sometimes about literature. Her daughter Lilah was born in July 2001.

Nikki Gemmell was born in Wollongong, Australia and is the author of the novels *Shiver*, *Cleave* and *Lovesong*. Her work has been internationally critically acclaimed and translated into many languages. She now lives in London with her husband and baby son.

David Guterson is the author of two novels, *Snow Falling on Cedars* and *East of the Mountains*, and a collection of short stories, *The Country Ahead of Us, the Country Behind*. He lives in Washington State, USA.

Kathryn Heyman grew up in Australia where she worked as an actor and playwright. Her novels are *The Breaking* (shortlisted for the Scottish Writer of the Year Award, longlisted for the Orange Prize) and *Keep Your Hands on the Wheel*. She has recently completed her third novel *The Accomplice*. After several years living in Scotland and Oxford, Kathryn is in the process, with her family, of moving back to Australia.

Nick Hornby was born in 1957, and is the author of four novels, *Fever Pitch*, *High Fidelity*, *About a Boy* and *How to be Good*. He is the pop music critic for the *New Yorker*, and in 1999 was awarded the E.M. Forster Award by the American Academy of Arts and Letters. He lives and works in Highbury, north London.

Alice Jerome was born in London in 1967, and has lived in Amherst, Massachusetts for the last five years with her husband and two daughters. She writes poetry and is currently working on a collection of novellas.

Simone Lazaroo was born in Singapore. She is the author

of two award-winning novels, *The World Waiting to be Made* (Fremantle Arts Centre Press) and *The Australian Fiancé* (Pan-Macmillan-Picador), and of various anthologised short stories. *The True Body* is part of a work in progress begun during her time as David T.K. Wong Fellow at the University of East Anglia. She currently teaches writing at Curtin University, Western Australia.

Chandani Lokugé came from Sri Lanka to Australia in 1987, on a Commonwealth Scholarship to read for a PhD in English, and is now lecturing at Monash University in Melbourne. She is the author of a novel, *If the Moon Smiled* (Penguin, 2000), shortlisted for NSW Premier's Award, and a collection, *Moth and Other Stories* (Aarhus: Dangaroo, 1994). Her short stories are widely anthologised including in *Penguin Summer Stories 3* (2000) and the *Penguin Anthology of Modern Sri Lankan Short Stories* (1998). She is currently editing a series of autobiographies and fiction written in English by Indian women for Oxford University Press. Her next novel, from which *Mala's Baby* is extracted, will be published by Penguin Australia in 2003.

Bridget O'Connor was born in London in 1961 to Irish parents. She is the author of two short-story collections, *Here Comes John* and *Tell Her You Love Her*, both published by Picador. She has also written a radio play, *Becoming the Rose*, broadcast on Radio Four and co-written two others under the title *The Centurions*. She currently lives in Hackney, east London with her partner and has one daughter.

Kathy Page's stories are widely anthologised, and collected in *As In Music* (Methuen). Her novels include *Back in the First Person* (Virago), *Island Paradise*, and *Frankie Styne and the Silver Man* (both Methuen). Her latest, *The Story of My Face*, was published by Weidenfeld and Nicolson in 2002, and another *Alphabet*, is forthcoming. She has recently moved from London to live on a small island off the west coast of Canada, with her husband and two children.

Emily Perkins was born in Christchurch, New Zealand in 1970 and grew up in Auckland and Wellington. She is a graduate of Bill Manhive's writing course at Victoria University, Wellington. She has published a collection of short stories, *Not Her Real Name*, and two novels, *Leave Before You Go* and *The New Girl*. She lives in London with her family.

Eva Sallis was born in Australia in 1964. Her first novel *Hiam* (Allen & Unwin, 1998) won the Australian/Vogel and the Dobbie Literary Awards. Her second novel *The City of Sealions* was published in 2002. Other publications include a book of literary criticism, *Sheherazade through the Looking Glass: the Metamorphosis of the 1001 Nights* (Curzon, 1999); and a number of short stories, poems, academic and literary articles, and reviews. She has a PhD specialising in comparative literature (Arabic and English) and is a lecturer in English at the University of Adelaide. She lives near Port Adelaide with her partner Roger and their son Rafael.

Polly Samson was born in London in 1962. Her collection of short stories *Lying in Bed* was published in 1999, followed by a novel *Out of the Picture*, both published by Virago. She is married with three sons and a daughter.

Rosie Waitt studied creative writing at the University of Technology in Sydney before moving to London. In 1997 she was awarded an MA in Writing from Sheffield Hallam University in the UK. Her fiction and travel writing have been published in anthologies and magazines in both the

UK and Australia. She now lives in Tasmania where she is juggling two projects: a novel, *The Curse* (helped along greatly by the receipt of a grant from Arts Tasmania), and a travel book *And Then There Were Five: A Year on the Road in Australia*.

# A NOTE ON THE TYPE

The text of this book is set in Linotype Sabon, named after the type founder, Jacques Sabon. It was designed by Jan Tschichold and jointly developed by Linotype, Monotype and Stempel, in response to a need for a typeface to be available in identical form for mechanical hot-metal composition and hand composition using foundry type.

Tschichold based his design for Sabon roman on a fount engraved by Garamond, and Sabon italic on a fount by Granjon. It was first used in 1966 and has proved an enduring modern classic.